# Discover Your Destiny With The Monk Who Sold His Ferrari

### The 7 Stages of Self-Awakening

## Robin Sharma

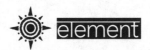

element

Element
An Imprint of HarperCollins*Publishers*
77–85 Fulham Palace Road,
Hammersmith, London W6 8JB

The website address is: www.thorsonselement.com

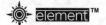

and *Element* are trademarks of
HarperCollins*Publishers* Ltd

First published by HarperCollins*Publishers* in 2004
This edition 2004

5 7 9 10 8 6 4

A catalogue record of this book
is available from the British Library

ISBN-13  978-0-00-719571-8
ISBN-10  0-00-719571-0

Printed and bound in Great Britain by
Creative Print and Design (Wales), Ebbw Vale

This book is dedicated to fellow seekers, those brave souls who exercise the courage to leave the crowd and find their way home to a place called authenticity.

May your resolve to awaken and live in *true* power be indomitable. May the lessons you are due to learn arrive in gentle ways. May your dark nights of the soul be few and far between. And may you shine so brightly that, at the end of your days, all will pause and say, "Ah, there was one who lived life fully and completely."

# Acknowledgements

I am blessed to be surrounded by many extraordinary people in my life. Without them, it would not be possible for me to do what I do and to advance my mission of helping people live their highest lives. For all who have helped in the shaping of my ideas, encouraged me to dream big dreams and aided in the spread of my message, I am deeply grateful.

I must offer special thanks to my team at Sharma Leadership International. In particular, thanks go to Marie Witten, my wonderful executive assistant; Al Moscardelli, whom I count on in so very many ways; and Marnie Ballane, whose enthusiasm always inspires me.

It is also important to express my gratitude to the entire HarperCollins team, which has been so supportive of my work. Thanks to Iris Tupholme, David Kent, Akka Janssen, Kevin Hanson, Noelle Zitzer, Lisa Zaritzky, Martha Watson, Lloyd Kelly, David Millar, Kristin Cochrane, Michaela Cornell, Neil Erickson, Alan Jones and Ian Murray, along with the account representatives who have helped get each of the books in *The Monk Who Sold His Ferrari* series out to my much-valued readers.

I also wish to acknowledge the outstanding work of my editor, Nicole Langlois, who has been with me from a very early point. You have been a true pleasure to work with on each occasion. Of course, I also must thank Sharma Leadership International's corporate clients who allow me the privilege of sharing my ideas on leadership, elite performance and self-mastery with your employees as a management consultant, executive coach and keynote speaker. I should say, as well, that I feel very fortunate to have the reader support that I do. All that I do, I do for the readers of my books, and I offer heartfelt thanks to each and every one of you for the belief you have in me. Thank you for giving me the chance to live my destiny.

My family has encouraged me from day one. When I had nothing but a self-published book and faced many closed doors, they offered me a foundation of inspiration and unforgettable support. I am blessed to have the parents that I have, two people whose wisdom and kindness have shaped me more than words can express. Thanks also to my brother Sanjay—a truly gifted human being—and to his wife, Susan, another wonderful person. I could not forget to note the gifts that their two great children, Neel and Evan, bring to my life. Special thanks to my sweetheart, Nina, for all your love and the blessings you have brought to me. And finally, I must acknowledge my two incredible children, Colby and Bianca, for teaching me the meaning of unconditional love, boundless creativity and genuine joy. You two bring so much wonder to my life, and I love you more than words can say.

*The hidden well-spring of your soul must needs rise and run murmuring to the sea;*
*And the treasure of your infinite depths would be revealed to your eyes.*
*But let there be no scales to weigh your unknown treasure;*
*And seek not the depths of your knowledge with staff or sounding line.*

Kahlil Gibran, *The Prophet*

*Gravedigger, when you dig my grave, could you make it shallow so that I can feel the rain.*

Dave Matthews, *Some Devil*

# An Introduction
# from Robin Sharma

*You are far greater than you have ever dreamed of being.* And no matter what you are experiencing in your life right now, trust that all is good and unfolding in your best interests. It may not look pretty, but it is exactly what you need to learn for you to grow into the person you have been destined to become. Everything occurring in your life has been perfectly orchestrated to inspire your maximal evolution as a human being and bring you into your true power. Learn from life and allow it to take you where you are meant to go—it has your highest interests in mind.

Within the pages of this book, you will discover many answers to life's most important questions. I pray you will find many truths and gain much insight into the way the world works and how you can succeed within it. But, ultimately, the answers you are seeking already lie deep within your heart. There is nowhere else to look. Yes, my words may prompt openings for you and serve to help you remember what you already know at your core. But do not doubt that there is, indeed, a treasure trove of wisdom, power and love slumbering within you—waiting to be awakened by your most courageous part. Isn't that incredibly inspiring to know? *You already are everything you have always wanted to become.* You simply need to do the inner work required to remove the blocks that have been covering—and denying—your original nature.

The purpose of human life, I believe, is to walk the path of this Great Awakening of Self and to return home to who you once were (and the place you once knew). My closely held belief is that newborn children represent perfection and the state of being to which each of us is duty-bound to return. In the instant after you were born, you were fearless, pure love, innocent, infinitely wise, of boundless potential and beautifully connected with the unseen hand that created the universe. As a very young child, you were filled with wonder and fully alive to life. Indeed, at that time you were nearly enlightened (to be enlightened is to be all light: one who is all light has no shadows, no dark side, no fears, no anger, no resentments and no limitations).

Most of us on the planet today have lost this connection to our authentic selves, this original state of being in which we were unafraid to walk towards possibility and reach for the stars. *We know not who we are.* We have morphed into people who behave selfishly, fearfully and hurtfully. This behavior is not a reflection of our essential nature but is, instead, a reflection of the wounds we have suffered as we have left the innocence to which we were born and traveled along the journey of our days. Only people in pain can do painful things. Only people who have been hurt can hurt others. Only people with closed hearts are able to act in less than loving ways.

The whole reason we are alive, I believe, is to grow into our greatest selves and *remember* the truth about who we fundamentally are. Life will support you perfectly in this quest. You will be sent people, events and trials that will invite you to reveal more of your brilliance and discover more of your possibilities. Often, your lessons will not come easily. Suffering has always been a vehicle for deep spiritual growth. Those who have endured great suffering are generally the ones who evolve into great beings. Those who have been deeply hurt by life are generally the ones who can feel the pain of others in a heartbeat. Those who have endured adversity become humbled by life, and as a result, are more open, compassionate and real. We may not like suffering when it visits us, but it serves us so very well: it cracks the shell that covers our hearts and empties us of the lies we have clung to about who we are, why we are here and how this remarkable world of ours really functions. Once emptied, we can be refilled with all that is good, noble and true. Troubles can transform, if we choose to allow them to do so. As Joseph Campbell wrote: "Where you stumble, there your treasure lies."

*Discover Your Destiny* is a book about reclaiming your greatest life. I have tried to pour my heart out onto these pages and share all I know about personal leadership, self-discovery and living from a place of authenticity. You should know that I am very human. I struggle daily with my limitations, my fears and what I call my "ancient patterns," those old ways of behaving that I have learned along the way. I see myself as a work in progress and continually challenge myself to use each day as a platform to evolve into the higher reaches of my inner life. There is a myth out there that people who write these kinds of books are enlightened beings who spend their days in bliss and transcendence, offering words of truth from the mountaintop. In reality, I have learned that every single one of us has work to do, no matter how much work we have done on ourselves, no matter how evolved we are. Every single one of us has a light side as well as a dark side. Each of us has flaws to mend and wounds within us that cry out to be healed. Every single one of us has a splintered soul (as we try to reconcile being spiritual with being human). This condition of imperfection is actually what makes us human. And the deeper I go within myself, the more I realize how little I know. As I wrote in *The Saint, The Surfer and The CEO*, "the top of one mountain is the bottom of the next." As we reach the summit of the mountain we are currently climbing, guess what we see? Other peaks to scale. This is what life on Schoolhouse Earth is all about: never-ending growth and learning that comes for the sole purpose (or should that be "soul purpose"?) of helping us remember and reclaim the greatness—and wholeness—that, sadly, we've lost.

And though I have my human limitations, I will also admit to you that I have come a long way in a short period of time in terms of removing the blocks that have kept me small (and so can you if you follow the extraordinary process explained on the pages that follow). Only a handful of years ago, I was a litigation lawyer on the fast-track to worldly success, chasing money, acclaim and materialism. I was living life from the outside in rather than from the inside out (no wonder it wasn't working). I endured a very hard divorce and now raise my two incredible children as a single father. Along the way, I suffered great setbacks and, at times, seemingly endless personal trials. *But we grow most from our greatest challenges.* I've realized that these experiences were sent to help me clean up my act and me to move through my weakness. Life's biggest hurts are, in truth, glorious opportunities for personal growth, positive transformation and reclaiming the authentic power you've lost as you left the perfection of infancy and walked into the world. Embrace them for the gifts they are.

Through all the highs and lows that this incredible (and short) game of life has sent my way, I have never given up on my commitment to accept responsibility for my part in all that has unfolded and to reach for my biggest self in the process. I believe that much of what we experience in life has been prescripted. But I also believe that we, as human beings, have an *enormous* amount of choice to create the beautiful lives of our dreams. Fate and our choices work in concert to sculpt the look of our lives. And it is in our conscious choice-making that, ultimately, our destinies are realized. To forget this is to play the victim. To disregard this truth is to deny the power that has been granted to you to create all that you want.

The pathway I've described in this book—The 7 Stages of Self-Awakening—reflects the eternal, archetypal journey of the leader or the hero. In the tradition of the previous books of *The Monk Who Sold His Ferrari* series, the messages in this book are revealed through the fictional adventures of Julian

Mantle. But it is important to remember that they are *very* real and exceptionally powerful. The process embodied within the seven stages can be found, in various forms, in many of the ancient texts of both Eastern and Western wisdom literature. You are the hero or heroine of your life. If you choose to play your biggest game as a human being (and I know you will), this is the path that you too must walk. Traveling it *guarantees* you authentic success.

The best way to learn is to teach. If you really want to own this material and integrate it into your life, it is *essential* that you teach it to someone within twenty-four hours of completing this book. This will serve two purposes: first, it will help you to integrate the knowledge; second, it will help those around you remember who *they* truly are. And as you read *Discover Your Destiny*, engage those you love in conversations about what you are learning. Share your insights. Put a voice to the changes you are committed to making in the move towards your greatest life. Doing so will deepen your conviction and generate results *that last*.

Thank you for picking up this book; I hope it delivers all you seek from it (and so much more). I am grateful that you would give me the hours of your life required to read and reflect upon this work. And I genuinely honor you for taking this *giant* step towards discovering your destiny. As you read this book and others in *The Monk Who Sold His Ferrari* series, you will be joining other women and men from around the world who have become part of a community. Extraordinary conversations happen at our gathering place, *robinsharma.com*, a site where you will find a wealth of tools and support as you walk the path of your destiny.

We are all connected at an invisible level. As you do your healing, you aid in the healing of the world. As you let your brilliance shine, you silently invite those around you to do the same. As you do the work required to let your life stand for the 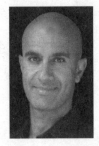 highest and the best, you serve as a model for others to play their highest game. And, as one of my coaching clients often says, "This is a beautiful thing."

I wish you immense blessings along this voyage called a life.


With Love,


Robin Sharma

# CHAPTER 1

A Spiritual Emergency

*Life does not listen to your logic; it goes on its own way, undisturbed. You have to listen to life; life will not listen to your logic, it does not bother about your logic.*

—Osho

I could feel the coolness of the metal against my head. How could it have come to this? I was actually sitting in a shabby motel room with a gun pushed up against my temple, ready to squeeze the trigger. Sweat was pouring down my forehead and my heart was beating wildly. My hands were shaking uncontrollably. No one knew where I was. No one seemed to care anymore. I had nothing to live for. So I was preparing to die.

I could see the headline of my obituary right now: "Dar Sandersen, international hotel entrepreneur, divorced father of three, dead at age 44—by his own hand."

But as I closed my eyes and said a final prayer aloud, something unexpected—no, miraculous—happened. I began to feel dizzy and fell to the floor, the gun dropping out of my hand. As I lay there, motionless, a blinding white light began to fill my body. But before you dismiss my story, please know that I've always been a very grounded and reasonable person. Nothing like this had ever happened to me before. I'd always chuckled on hearing stories of the mystical, deeming them flaky and irresponsible. I didn't—and still don't—talk to angels, nor do I run my life according to the daily position of the stars. Yet, I cannot discount or deny what happened to me in that motel room only twelve months ago. Was it an experience of the divine? Was it a spiritual awakening? Was it simply a physical reaction to the extreme stress I was experiencing? Truthfully, I do not know. What I do know is what happened there set into motion a series of events that have transformed every element of the life I once knew.

The light grew brighter and brighter. Soon, my entire body began to shake, as if I were experiencing a massive seizure. Sweat flowed out of me in torrents as my arms, legs and torso trembled on the cold and filthy floor. This continued for what seemed like an eternity. Then, seemingly out of nowhere, came these words that pierced the deepest part of me: *"Your life is a treasure and you are so much more than you know."*

That was it. Once these words flashed across my mind, I stopped shaking. I just lay there, in a pool of perspiration, staring up at the ceiling. I had never felt such internal peace in all my life. I was completely in my body, fully within my heart. *Life is a treasure and you are so much more than you know.*

After a while, I slowly rose to my feet and packed up my belongings. Something deep within me had shifted, though I can't explain it—I just *felt* it. I no longer had an interest in taking my own life. Maybe that voice was right—maybe I did have much more within me than I was currently aware of.

Generally, when we face hard times, we think the way we see

the world reflects the way it really is. This is a false assumption. We are simply viewing the world from our hopeless frame of reference. We are seeing things through sad and hopeless eyes. The truth of the matter is that when we begin to feel better, our world will look better. And when we return to a state of joyfulness within, our outer world will reflect that feeling to us. I've learned that the world is a mirror. *We receive from life not what we want but who we are.* I've also learned that there are seasons to our lives and painful times never last. *Trust that the winter of your sorrow will yield to the summer of your joy, just as the brilliant rays of the morning always follow the darkest part of the night.*

I no longer was a desperate case, feeling sorry for myself. I no longer saw no way out. Some sort of power had been returned to me that day. And though my life was still a mess, truth be told, I had begun to know that I possessed the power to improve it. For some reason, *I trusted* that help was on the way and that happier days were coming. Little did I know how wonderful this help would be and how beautiful my life would become. But before I get into these details, you may be wondering what circumstances led my spirit to fall into such a state of decay that I could even consider taking my own life.

Only a few years ago, I thought I was living the life everyone dreamed of. I had a lovely and intelligent wife who loved me deeply. I had three healthy and happy children who excelled at all they chose to do. I was making more money than I could have ever imagined, as the owner of a string of hip boutique hotels located at sophisticated hot spots around the globe. Movie stars, the fabulously wealthy and the glitterati in general were among my clients. I traveled to exotic places, accumulated many toys and became fairly well known, at least in the marketspace within which I worked.

Then, one day, my entire world fell apart. I arrived home late after a business dinner with the vendor of a property I was interested in buying. Rachel usually left a few lights on for me but, on this night, the house was completely dark. It made no sense—it was only ten o'clock. Where was Rachel? Where were the kids?

I walked inside and turned on the lights in the entrance hall and the kitchen. Only silence greeted me. But on the kitchen table was a note in Rachel's familiar handwriting. It read:

*Dar, I've taken the kids to my mother's place. I do not love you anymore. I'm sorry. My lawyer will call you in the morning.*

Nothing can prepare you for a letter like that—nothing. Although I had pretended that my marriage was working, I knew we had drifted apart. All the time away from home, traveling and doing business, had been time stolen away from my marriage and family, and the love we once knew was gone. I had also pretended to be a good father and, from the outside, I probably seemed that. But the wise souls of my children knew the truth. Even when I was sitting right next to them, I wasn't really there. My mind never left the business and emotionally, I was unavailable. I guess the truth is that I was an extraordinarily selfish man back then. I believed the world revolved around me. No one else's needs and no one else's feelings mattered nearly as much as mine. I wanted to be rich. I wanted to be recognized. I wanted to win. And in the process, I lost what was most important.

The letter and the divorce litigation that ensued ripped my heart out. I was forced out of my own home and began to live in one of my hotels. I could see my kids only once a week and every few weekends. I began to drink heavily and gained an embarrassingly excessive amount of weight. I had always been ruggedly handsome and very fit, but that all unraveled. I'd wake up with searing migraines that would not leave me until I doused them with alcohol. Thankfully, I did not lose my business. I'd been smart enough to put in place a first-class management team who, out of loyalty to me, ran the show while I was busy licking my wounds. Sure, I'd attend the odd meeting and close the odd deal. But, mostly, I was home alone, sitting in a dark room listening to old Billie Holiday songs and having long conversations with Jack Daniels. This was the misery that eventually led me to that seedy motel room I told you about. But you should know that this was the misery that also led to my salvation.

I have discovered that pain and adversity are powerful vehicles to promote personal growth. Nothing helps you learn, grow and evolve more quickly. Nothing offers you as big an opportunity to reclaim more of your authentic power as a person. Our human eyes view it as a negative experience. This is pure *judgment* and behind this false belief is pure fear. You see, suffering occurs when something happens that we did not want. It occurs when life gives us something unexpected, some new condition. And the appearance of a new condition in our lives, whether this means an illness or the loss of a loved one or a financial setback, means we must change and leave the old, the shores we once clung to. We are asked to let go of what we expected and, for a human being, letting go can be frightening.

We are afraid to leave the safe harbor of the familiar and the known. We resist traveling to the unknown places our lives sometimes lead us towards. The very thought of doing so scares us. Behind all resistance to the new is fear.

*But there is nothing to fear.* This universe of ours is a far friendlier place than we realize. A boat that never ventures beyond its moorings will never be damaged, but that's not what boats are made for. Similarly, a human being who never dares to walk out into the unknown spaces of his or her life will never get hurt—but that is not what human beings were designed for. We were made to experience the growth that comes from visiting foreign places as travelers through life. Our wiser eyes know this truth and see change and suffering for what it really is: a caring physician that comes to heal the sick part of our selves. Suffering serves to deepen us. Suffering comes to help us and causes us to know who we truly are. Suffering cracks us open, forcing us to let go and surrender all that we have known and clung to, like a little child on her first day of school, afraid to let go of her mother's hand and walk alone into a classroom full of new friends where she will learn so many new and beautiful things. The unknown is where "the new" exists and the new is the only place in the world where you will find *possibility*. And every human being is hardwired to run towards possibility and potential in their lives. We were all designed to be great. So how can you say suffering is bad when it is the very thing that makes you better? Yes, the human side of us feels the pain as we endure it. That's natural. But this pain will eventually subside and a richer, stronger, wiser you will emerge.

*"Fear not the unknown, for it is where your greatness*

*resides,*" said a very special teacher of mine, one whom you are about to learn much about. Most people spend the best years of their lives in the place of the known. They lack the courage to venture out into foreign territory and are frightened to leave the crowd. They want to fit in and are afraid to stand out. They dress like everyone else, think like everyone else and behave like everyone else, even if doing so doesn't feel right to them. They are reluctant to listen to the call of their hearts and try new things, refusing to leave that shore of safety. So they do what everybody else does. In so doing, their once-shining souls begin to darken and wrinkle. "Death is only one of many ways to lose your life," said adventurer Alvah Simon.

Clinging to safe shores in your life is nothing more than making a choice to remain imprisoned by your fears. There may be the illusion that you are free when you keep living within the box that your life may have become but, believe me, it's just that: an illusion—a lie you tell yourself. When you leave the box for new vistas and stop following the crowd, of course, fears will surface—you are human. But courage requires that you feel these fears and then move ahead any-way. *Courage is not the absence of fear but the willingness to walk through your fear in pursuit of a goal that is important to you.* You are among the living dead when you live in a safe harbor and cling to the known. You come back to life and your heart starts to beat again when you venture into the unknown and explore the foreign places of your life. The adventure and thrill of living returns. *Remember, on the other side of your fears you will discover your fortune.*

Here's a strong metaphor I'll offer you. If you have spent your whole life in a jail, many fears will surface on the day of your release. While in jail, though you had no freedom, you lived within the realm of the known because there was a strict routine in place for you: you knew when you were required to wake, you knew when you could exercise and you knew precisely when and what you could eat. Now, though you are no longer imprisoned, you feel afraid. You do not know what to do and where to go. There is no structure, only uncertainty. Your tendency is to return to the known rather than face the seeming insecurity and discomfort of the unknown. You would rather choose to be a prisoner than regain your freedom. It makes no sense but that's how most of us operate through life.

I have learned all this philosophy from the teacher I briefly mentioned. This teacher has been the single greatest influence on my life to date. The wisdom and the remarkable seven-stage process he began to share with me just over twelve months ago have completely revolutionized my life. I have never been so happy. I have never felt so alive. I have never had so much self-respect. I have found the love of my life. My health is perfect. And my business is soaring. I never imagined life could be this good. The same can hold true for you. The gifts I've received are gifts available to you as well. Sure, you will have to make some new choices and take a few chances. Sure, you will have to invest some time and energy to reconnect with the great and magnificent parts of yourself that you may have lost. Sure, you may have to face a few fears that have been keeping you small, whether you've acknowledged it or not. But in so doing you will awaken your highest and greatest self. And what could possibly be more important than that?

The teacher I've mentioned is the wisest, most powerful and

most noble person I know. He is an eccentric—a true original—and his ways are unorthodox, to put it mildly. Actually, he's a bit of a wildman at times. You have never met anyone like him and you never will. But he is so very gifted in his ability to impart life-altering knowledge in a way that speaks to your soul and causes you to experience changes that will open up a beautiful life for you. His lessons will be very helpful as you seek to discover your destiny and live the gorgeous life that is your birthright.

I guess there are no accidents. I met my teacher the day after my epiphany in the motel room. I went to work that day for a meeting with my team, and my human resources manager, Evan Janssen, walked into my office with two tickets to a motivational seminar later that evening. Evan loved these kinds of events and was a huge fan of the whole personal growth movement. I, on the other hand, was a skeptic. To be honest with you, I don't like motivational speakers at all. I've always found them to be a bit like cotton candy—sweet for a few moments but you soon discover that nothing lasts.

Evan's little boy had his first piano recital that night, so Evan couldn't attend the seminar. He wanted me to go. He thought the event would lift my spirits and perhaps inspire me to make the changes in my life he knew I needed to get back on track, not only professionally but personally. I told him I didn't want to go and just couldn't stomach the trite aphorisms and clichéd homilies commonly recited by motivators. I mentioned that I was still struggling with a lot of things and felt it best to be alone that evening. Then something interesting happened. My colleague, a highly intuitive man, looked deep into my eyes and said, "Dar, trust me on this one. I feel there is a reason you need to go to this seminar. It's just a feeling I have in my gut. *Please* go."

I have always been a man who lived mostly in his head. Reason rather than passion drove me. If something didn't make sense at an intellectual level, I'd usually discount it. But I'd lived that way my whole life and my life still wasn't working. I love Einstein's definition of insanity: "Doing the same things and expecting different results." If I wanted new results in my life I knew I had to behave in *new* ways. Otherwise my life would look the same, until I died.

Something deep within me suggested that there just might be another way to operate as a human being. I had recently read my very first book of philosophy, though I had never touched that kind of thing before. I don't know what compelled me to pick it up but I did. Maybe, being in so much pain, I was ready to look anywhere for salvation. *It is a truth that in our darkest times we are willing to go the deepest.* When life is good, we live superficially; we are not very reflective. But when the seas get rough, we step out of ourselves and ponder why things have unfolded as they have. Adversity tends to make us more philosophical. During times of challenge, we begin to ask ourselves the bigger questions of life, such as why does suffering happen, why do our best-laid plans not work out as we expect, and is life ruled by the silent hand of chance or the powerful fist of choice.

In this book I picked up, the author wrote that the mind is limited while the heart is limitless. The mind can be cruel, causing you to spend the best years of your life living in the past or squandering the present worrying over things that will never happen. The mind craves *external* power, the kind based on worldly—rather than spiritual—things such as money, position and possessions. The problem with external power is that it is fleeting: when you lose the money, position and possessions, you lose the power. If you have tied your identity to those things, you will also lose a sense of who you are when they fall away. The only power worth anything is authentic power—that which comes from within.

The heart, according to this book, has no desire for these minor pursuits. The heart lives in the present moment, knowing that is where life is to be lived. The heart is concerned with healing into wholeness, love, compassion and service to other human beings. It is aware that each of us is connected at an unseen level, that we are all brothers and sisters of the same family and that happiness comes from giving and supporting the growth of others into their greatest selves. "Give up the drop, become the ocean," said the brilliant Sufi poet Rumi. The heart knows this truth. Yes, the mind, with all its ability to reason and reflect, is a great *tool* that the heart should use to support its work, a tool that can be used for things like planning, learning and thinking. But these functions must be done in concert with the heart, and under its guidance. The head and heart must forge a lifetime *partnership* if one wants to live a beautiful life, the book informed me. They must work in *harmony*. Live completely in the head and you cannot *feel* the breath and rhythm of life. Live completely in the heart and you may find yourself acting like a love-struck fool, with poor judgment and no discipline. It's all a fine balance, one that takes time, energy and understanding to get right.

Standing there, with Evan waiting patiently, I felt a pull to explore something new. Taking a moment to pay attention to what was happening below the surface, I decided to let go of the limitations of reason for a while and trust my deeper feelings. I agreed to go and took the tickets.

Evan reached over and gave me a hug. "We love you, you know."

I was quiet as emotion welled up inside me on hearing this statement of profound kindness from my long-time colleague. Tears began to flow, partly over the sadness I felt from the way my life had unfolded in recent times and partly from the unconditional love I felt from another human being.

"Thanks, Evan," I replied. "You're a good man. I appreciate you."

"Trust me, Dar, this seminar's going to be really important for you. And who knows who you'll meet there?"

Little did I know, I was about to meet the man who would lead me to my greatest life.

# CHAPTER 2

# The Seeker Meets a Master

*We shall not cease from exploration. And the end of
all our exploring will be to arrive where we started
and know the place for the first time.*

—T. S. Eliot

That night found me sitting in a room with five thousand other
people seeking the answers to life's biggest questions. Rock
music blared from the speakers and a dazzling light show lit
up the otherwise dark and cavernous room. There was a pal-
pable energy in the room. Then the speaker emerged. He was
handsome, articulate and extremely charismatic. He spoke
eloquently and kept the audience's rapt attention for nearly
two hours as he took us on an emotional roller coaster that
made us laugh, cry and think about why we lived as we did and
how each one of us could make things better. He talked about
his childhood growing up without a father. He discussed his
brush with cancer and how it helped connect him to the sim-
pler, yet commonly neglected things in life. And he made us
laugh at some of his insights, such as "the only thing you can
expect in life is the unexpected" and "if you want to make God
laugh, tell him your plans." I also appreciated his humility. He

said he was not a guru but simply a student of life and joked that his morning prayer involved the request: "God, please help me to become the person my dog thinks I am."

"*Your wounds must be turned into your wisdom,*" he repeated throughout the presentation. "Your stumbling blocks can become your stepping stones *if you choose*. Do not miss the remarkable opportunity that adversity and even tragedy presents. *Your life can be made even better by the things that break your heart.*"

By the end of his speech, the speaker had each of his listeners spellbound. There was utter silence as we hung on his every word. He closed his presentation with the following statement: "Most people don't discover how to live until it's time to die—and that's a shame. Most people spend the best years of their lives watching television in a subdivision. Most people die at twenty and are buried at eighty. *Please*, don't let that happen to you."

After receiving a thunderous standing ovation, the speaker left the stage. I just sat there silently as question after question began to surface in my mind. "Why was I feeling so empty in life?" No matter how much money I made or how successful I became, I still didn't feel any differently. I also wondered whether my chosen career was the one I was supposed to be doing or if there was something else that was destined to be my "life work." As well, I questioned whether I would find true love in my life and whether soul mates could really exist. It was interesting to me that so many questions began to arise once I took just a little bit of time to be silent and still.

As I dug deeper, more questions surfaced: Did I have choice as to how my life unfolded or was it all predetermined according to some grand master plan? If I did have choice, what was keeping me from taking steps to make things better? Was there truly a better life waiting for me out there or was that just wishful thinking? I also wondered whether everything that had happened between Rachel and me had been orchestrated by some invisible force of nature or whether the way things unfolded for us was nothing more than a reflection of my personal choices: to put my business ahead of my family, to put my needs first, to do whatever I wanted to do instead of being big-hearted, compassionate and caring. I closed my eyes and thought about these important questions. I then did something I had never done before: I began to pray for answers.

After only a few minutes, I heard someone call out my name. I looked around but, oddly, I couldn't see anyone I recognized. Given the traumatic experience of the night before, I wondered whether I was going crazy. Only twenty-four hours earlier I had experienced white light flooding through my body and received the message *"Life is a treasure and you are so much more than you know,"* and now I was hearing my name being called out in a near-empty auditorium after an unforgettable motivational seminar. I closed my eyes once more—only to hear my name being called again! I quickly opened my eyes and looked around, but again, I could see no one I knew. This time, though, I saw a strange but unmistakable clue on the chair next to mine: a crisp white envelope, with my name inscribed in elegant red handwriting. It had been sealed. I ripped it open and read the words on the page: "Stop living your life as a lie, Dar. Be true to yourself and your destiny will come knocking. I'll meet you backstage. Nice shirt, by the way—I like the stripes, very hip."

What was going on? Evan had told me something important would happen at this motivational rally, but this was bordering on the surreal. My heart started beating quickly, and I wondered if this was a practical joke or if I was perhaps being drawn into a dangerous situation. But something within me had been stirred by the motivational speaker's presentation, as if he had planted some seeds that were already beginning to germinate. One word quickly came to my mind: *trust*. I picked up my notes and put them into my Gucci briefcase. I then stood up and, not without reservation, walked to the edge of the stage from which the speaker had delivered his inspirational performance. I made my way to the curtains near the front of the stage and slipped through an opening in the folds of fabric.

Backstage, all was a flurry of activity. The speaker was not in sight, but the audiovisual technicians were hard at work, packing equipment into aluminum boxes. No one seemed to notice me. As I continued walking around the backstage area, a door slowly opened, allowing a bright light to emerge and illuminate the dimly lit area. I felt as if I was being guided towards that door, odd as that may sound. I literally felt *pulled* in the direction of that door; I moved through it and into a hallway. My heart was beating rapidly and my stomach was knotted with anxiety as I walked down the hall. I felt shaky and uncertain. But I also felt a confidence I had not previously encountered, one that gently suggested to me that somehow things were taken care of.

The hallway led to a red door with nothing but a silver star on it. I guessed that this was the dressing room reserved for the stars who gave performances in this auditorium. I knocked three times on the door. No one answered. I knocked again, with more vigor. Again, there was no response. I waited for a few moments and then decided that maybe I was wasting my time. The note had instructed me to go backstage but no one was here. It all made no sense. I was feeling tired and was in serious need of some sleep. It had been a rough two days and a hot cup of tea might soothe my frazzled nerves.

I was about to turn away when, as if by magic, the door opened. I couldn't see anyone behind the door but the door continued to open wider. As I stepped into the room, I was *stunned* by what I saw. Rose petals had been strewn across the floor. A tall figure stood before me wearing a scarlet robe, the kind worn by monks in Nepal. His back was facing me and he stood motionless. The intricate embroidery on the back of his robe caught my eyes. It was beautiful and rich with color. For some reason, I began to relax and let out a sigh. I felt— don't ask me why—that I was in the presence of a friend.

Slowly and dramatically, the figure turned towards me and looked straight into my eyes. He seemed to touch my soul with his striking gaze. In my entire life, I have never met anyone who exuded such power. He looked youthful, tanned, had a thick head of dark hair and seemed to be in superb physical condition, looking like some Greek god from a bygone era or, perhaps, a movie star from Hollywood. And his eyes! I will never forget those eyes. They were the most piercing and remarkable eyes I have ever seen.

Who was this man? Why was he staring at me? Why wasn't I afraid? I didn't know what to do and just stood there, awestruck by the entire experience. The room remained silent and this stranger remained motionless and without expression.

Then his mouth curved in a gentle smile and his eyes began to sparkle like a child's. He spoke in a confident tone.

"Only you can discover your destiny, Dar. Only you can know the path that has been laid out for you, the one your heart is calling you to walk. But having a guide will make the journey easier—we all need a good life coach to help us reach our biggest lives. The Zen sages say that when the student is ready, the teacher will appear. Now, that phrase may be over-used, but it also happens to be true. I'm so happy that you trusted your instincts and came here tonight. You don't need to be afraid. I know what's happened to you. I know of your loss. I know of your suffering. I know of your confusion. I also know something of your longings."

"My longings? What do you mean?" I asked in a quiet voice.

"You are a seeker, as are so many others on the planet today. The world is transforming as people who were once willing to live ordinary lives now step out of their comfort zones to explore the wilderness of the extraordinary. People are no longer willing to settle for being half-alive, divorced from their authentic power. They want to live greatly and soar among the clouds, to walk among the giants, to dance with the stars!" His forceful voice rose passionately to fill the small room.

Now he began to laugh. What a heartfelt and contagious laugh!

"Forgive me, Dar, I'm getting a little carried away. It's just that I am so excited about what's happening in the world today. Millions and millions of people are standing up for their best lives. So many people are refusing to play the victim and instead choosing to play the victor. So many people are going deep within themselves to visit and conquer their fears.

Hearts are opening right across the globe and people are reclaiming the brilliant and wonderful parts of themselves that they lost as they grew up and became adults. It's an extraordinary time to be alive. The whole world is becoming a better place to be. Actually, there's never been a better time to be a human being."

"It doesn't seem like it to me," I offered, the skeptic in me coming to the surface. "There are wars, famine, crime. Our environment is in a mess. Don't get me wrong, I'm not the most socially conscious guy out there, but even I can see that the world is a very uncertain and turbulent place."

"Quite true," the man replied with humility, as if he had nothing to prove to me, no ego investment in appearing right. "There is still much darkness in the world. But, trust me, there is also more light in it than ever. So many people have come to realize that you can curse the darkness or you can have the courage to be one who lights a candle. That's what leadership as a human being is all about—lighting candles amidst darkness. Darkness only exists in the absence of light. And candles are being lit all across the planet, metaphorically speaking. We are moving towards a critical mass, a tipping point when there will be a massive shift. It's not so far away. When enough people awaken to who they truly are and reclaim their highest potential, there will be a quantum leap. This whole world will be a lovely place to be—Heaven on Earth."

"Heaven on Earth? A quantum leap?"

"Yes. There will be a quantum leap in the numbers of people who will be on the path to authenticity—a path that involves living life on your own terms, according to your deepest values and highest ideals. It's a path that involves living with a wide open heart and a well-developed mind. It's a path that's all about confronting your fears and the things that keep you small so you can let your bigness shine. It's beautiful, baby!" the stranger said with a wink.

"There will be a quantum leap in the numbers of people who will be willing to heal their shadow sides and never do anything to hurt or limit another person. There will be a quantum leap in the numbers of people who will refuse to live a life that is less than noble, good and fearless. There will be a quantum leap in the numbers of people who will assume genuine *leadership* over their lives. There will be a quantum leap in the number of people who will become seekers, just like you, Dar, searching for happiness, inner peace and a life of deep meaning. There is a huge evolutionary shift occurring for humankind. The whole species is changing. We are refusing to accept anything less than personal greatness," he added enthusiastically.

"What do you mean by an 'evolutionary shift'?"

"Thanks for asking. There are no silly questions in this important conversation, you know. Most of our evolution, as human beings, to date has been marked by a focus on the physical, on the external. It has, until now, all been about accumulation and hoarding. The dominant value has been 'he who has the most wins'—he who has the most fame, he who has the biggest fortune, he who wields the most power over others. And given this value, 'survival of the fittest' has become the name of the game. It's all about competition because we have come to believe that there is not enough for everyone to win. But this philosophy no longer serves us as a race. It is one born of scarcity. And behind this thought of scarcity is out-right fear. Since our intentions and what we think create what we see in our outer world, all we see is lack—there's never enough for us. And so the cycle begins, we never feel as if we have enough and we are never happy."

"Fascinating. I've never heard anything like this," I remarked, sitting down on a chair in the dressing room. The stranger remained standing with his hands folded behind him.

"Now here's what I mean by the 'evolutionary shift': many human beings on the planet are taking their focus away from the single-minded concern over the physical and paying far more attention to the spiritual. We are moving from indepen-dence, where it's all about 'me, me, me' to an appreciation for the paramount importance of 'interdependence.' Many of us have become conscious of the fact that we are all part of the same family. The most evolved among us in the world today, the *authentic* leaders—and by leaders I do not necessarily mean CEOs, presidents and military generals, but all women and men who have refused to follow the crowd—have realized that, at the deepest level, we are all connected. They know that when you hurt another, you are really hurting yourself. They know that when you help another, you are really helping yourself. Even frontier science is now showing this, confirming empiri-cally what the mystics have been saying for thousands of years. Quantum physicists have discovered that the universe is a stun-ningly interconnected system where everything is in relation-ship with—and affected by—everything else. The English poet John Donne was speaking truth when he wrote: "No man is an island, entire of itself; every man is a piece of the continent, a part of the main . . . any man's death diminishes me, because I am involved in mankind; and therefore never send to know for whom the bell tolls; it tolls for thee."

"This is very interesting," I replied, truly engaged in this new information I was hearing.

"So many of us have shifted our focus from a quest for the external to a voyage into the internal. For many, the human journey has become an inner journey. We have realized that the gateway to lasting success does not swing outward, it opens inward. *The greatest treasures are the treasures that lie within.* We, as a species, are now beginning to think far more about the needs of our souls and devoting more time to activities like personal growth, being more loving and compassionate and leaving a legacy. *Success is important but significance is even better.* Just look at the books on the bestseller lists around the world—so many of them are about the quest for self-knowledge and personal freedom. People all over the planet, in masses, are asking the big questions of life, such as 'why am I here?' and 'what is my destiny?' And, as I say, the more people change, the more the whole world will change. It's a very beautiful process that's taking place. And it really is an exquisite time to be alive."

"That's very inspiring," I noted, relaxing even more and fully absorbing what I was hearing. I unfolded my arms.

"Now don't get me wrong," said the monk. "There's nothing wrong with making money, having nice things and living a physically beautiful life. We are spiritual beings having a human experience and life can be made better through enjoying the wonderful things human beings have created. Money makes life easier and affords a great deal of freedom. Anyone who tells you otherwise is probably suffering from the Ostrich Syndrome."

"What's that?"

"Too many people avoid dealing with the truth. It's easier to stick your head in the sand like an ostrich than confront your resistances to the truth. And the truth of the matter is that there's absolutely nothing wrong with making money and having beautiful things. Who came up with the silly notion that you cannot have nice things and, at the same time, be spiritual, good and evolved anyway? Have a lovely home. Drive a fine car. Travel to exotic places. Wear beautiful clothes. I'm *not* suggesting that you do not experience and enjoy such worldly pleasures. Ultimately, these were created by the same hidden force that created the streams, the mountains and the trees. But remember that beauty is only skin deep. These things must not be your driving force. Do not base your identity and your self-worth on them. Know that they will not last. It's more a matter of priorities—do not make the accumulation of such external things your primary priority. We come into the world with nothing and we leave with nothing. I've never seen a U-haul following a hearse on the way to a cemetery. That's the key thing to remember. *Have your beautiful things but do not be imprisoned by them. Own them but do not let them own you. Give the main aim of your life over to far more important pursuits such as discovery of your highest potential, giving of yourself to others and making a difference by living for something more important than yourself. Success is fine but significance is the real name of the game,"* he re-emphasized.

All of this man's wisdom was exactly what I needed to hear at this juncture of my life. Perhaps I really was the student and perhaps I had finally arrived at a place where I was ready to learn, and now the teacher appeared. Maybe nothing I had experienced in my life up to this point was a waste. Maybe it was all meant to be—all preparation to get me to this point of readiness. Evan, my human resources manager—a very spiritual man—frequently used the phrase "all is well in the universe" whenever something did not go as planned. No matter what unfolded for him at work and in life he'd say that it was "all good," even when it was painful. I was getting the sense that he was speaking truthfully. Perhaps there really were no accidents and the intricacies of our lives all happened according to a subtle yet perfect intelligence that, try as we might, we could not understand.

"I hope you don't mind my asking, but who are you?" I asked, mustering up my courage and hoping not to offend, in any way, this peculiar yet unforgettable man who was sharing his profound wisdom with me.

"My name is Julian Mantle and I have come to serve as your guide. I'm here to help you discover your destiny," came the simple reply.

He then reached into a wide silk pocket that had been sewn into his robe and pulled out a banana. Can you believe that? A banana! He peeled it and began munching away on it contentedly.

"Want one?" he asked graciously. "I have another in my knapsack," he said, pointing to a tattered canvas bag in the corner. "Bananas are excellent fuel for the body. The body must be nourished with only the best foods if you want it to perform at its highest level."

I hardly heard what he said—my mind started racing.

Julian Mantle! Unbelievable! I knew who Julian Mantle was. *Everyone* I knew recognized the name of Julian Mantle. I could not contain my excitement.

"Julian Mantle! The Monk Who Sold His Ferrari? Are you serious?" The whole scene felt surreal: the monk in front of me, the wise words he had offered, the chomping of the banana. It was as though I was having an out-of-body experience, watching the whole thing unfold from above. Yesterday I had a gun to my head, ready to take my life. Only one day later, I'm hanging out backstage after a motivational seminar with an eccentric monk who is telling me about the value of banana-eating and sharing his thoughts on the spiritual transformation that is occurring across the planet. Simply unbelievable.

I had heard about Julian on a regular basis since I was young. My father was a litigation lawyer who worked with one of the largest firms in the city and he would constantly entertain me with stories of "the great Julian Mantle." Julian was one of the nation's best trial lawyers and a man who was known far and wide not only for his abundant legal gifts but also for his high-flying, jet-set lifestyle. Julian Mantle was a superstar in the truest sense of the word. He had everything a human being could want. But he threw it all away.

Julian had graduated from Harvard Law School and was destined for a life of success. He was a "golden boy" and seemed unstoppable as he attracted the biggest cases, the best clients and scored win upon win. Along the way, he made more money than my father ever imagined a lawyer making and gained more publicity in one month than most lawyers generated over their entire careers. Dad said he dated the most beautiful women in the city, mostly fashion models, and was loved by all for his larger-than-life persona and roguish charm. When I was younger, my dad would drive me through the most posh area of the city and point out Julian's sprawling mansion, which sat only a few doors down from the home of one of the world's most famous rock stars. Julian appeared to live fully and to have it all. He even had a bright red Ferrari that he used to park in the center of his driveway. I still remember how much I loved looking at that car as a boy. I would have given anything for a ride in it. Dad said it was Julian's most loved possession.

And then something happened to Julian Mantle, according to my dad. He began to unravel. He gained weight and started to smoke too much. He began taking too many chances and lost too many cases. I wasn't really sure what caused this undoing but it was the most striking fall from grace that any one of us had ever seen. I guess the higher you go, the harder you fall. And then one day, in the middle of a packed courtroom amidst a particularly high-profile trial, Julian collapsed, apparently of a heart attack. My dad told me that that was the defining moment of Julian Mantle's life— the turning point. How we show up when we meet the turning points of our lives has a big influence on how our lives ulti- mately unfold, I have learned. What Julian did next altered the course of his life forever.

After months of recuperation, Julian resigned from the practice of law and left the country. He sold his mansion. Sold his possessions. He even sold his prized Ferrari as he departed for India, that exotic land of a million adventures and timeless wisdom. My guess is that he was looking for some answers and that India seemed to offer him some promise of finding them. No one heard from Julian for a long, long time. Many thought he was dead.

A number of months ago I read a front-page article entitled *"Julian Mantle: The Monk Who Sold His Ferrari. One Man's Crusade to Improve the World."* The article revealed that Julian Mantle had undergone a remarkable transformation while he was in India. High in the Himalayas, he had discovered a little-known group of monks. They had shared with him an ancient and profound philosophy for personal transformation and living one's greatest life. Through the extraordinary wisdom he learned, Julian experienced massive—and wonderful—changes in his own life. Physically, he recreated himself so that he looked many years younger than his actual age, exuding a vitality that was truly exceptional. Intellectually, he accessed the most universal truths upon which a rich and meaningful life is built and integrated them into the way he viewed the world, finding inner peace in the process. Emotionally, he became aware of many of the wounds that he had suffered during his childhood, wounds that were still running his life as an adult and blocking him from experiencing the joys that each one of us deserves to experience on a daily basis. This then allowed him to clear much of the anger he had been carrying with him through life, affecting him physically and psychically. He was able to heal the hurts of the past. Spiritually, he accessed his deepest values and reconnected with his highest self. Julian took off the social mask he had been wearing his whole life and became authentic, now living his life on *his* own terms, congruent with *his* highest values and according to the dictates of *his* heart. He stopped living to please others and stopped caring about looking good in the world. He refused to follow the crowd and betray himself, in any way. All he cared about now was *being real and doing good.* "Julian Mantle has discovered his destiny and this has made him a very happy man," I recalled the account stating.

The article also said that Julian had made it his central mission to come back to the West and help as many other people as he could to live their best lives and access the fullness of their potential. The story explained how Julian had been popping up, in his red robes, at different places and helping some of his old friends, family members and strangers reclaim their personal greatness and live far happier, healthier and fulfilling lives. The reporter wrote that Julian's work was creating an enormous buzz and that many people across the country were starting to put together expeditions to seek him out. Julian had become a folk hero of sorts and a mystique had begun to arise around him. But Julian was remarkably elusive: no person who had actively searched for Julian had been able to find him. Julian had not been interviewed in the story, but many had started calling him "The Reluctant Guru." The tale of Julian's life would have made for a fabulous movie in this age when so many of us are so spiritually starved.

"Are you really Julian Mantle?" I asked, still not quite believing. "Why did you come looking for me? My dad used to tell me about you. He was one of your colleagues, you know."

"I know *exactly* who your father is," came the gentle reply. "He was a friend of mine, and I value my friendships enormously. Your dad told me a lot about you, and I heard about what happened to your family life recently. I've come to be of service. Servant leaders are the most powerful of all, you know."

"Never knew that," I responded.

*"Things are never as bad as they seem. The situations that cause us sorrow are the same ones that introduce us to the strength, power and wisdom that we truly are."*

He continued. "I know things have been extremely difficult for you, Dar. I am very sensitive to what you are going through and I would never minimize your feelings. *Feelings are the doorways into your soul and they must be acknowledged and then felt to completion. Feelings carry important information and serve to foster your self-relationship if explored fully.* To deny them is to deny a natural part of you. To pretend you are not feeling what you are feeling would be a very unhealthy thing to do, both psychologically and physiologically. Swallowing your feelings leads to dis-ease. But there is a much bigger picture at play, one that you cannot comprehend with your current perception. Remember, we see the world not as it is but as we are. As you change, the way you see the world changes. *As your awareness expands, you will become aware of things you previously could neither see nor understand.* All is good here. All that has unfolded for you is leading you to a fantastic place. As human beings, our tendency is to tell life to listen to what we want. But life doesn't work that way. It gives us what we need, what is best for us—what is in our highest interests. *Your life will work much better once you begin to listen to life. Let it lead you rather than trying to push the river. And trust that where life carries you is exactly where you are meant to be. Let go of all your resistance and move into a posture of surrendering to whatever is unfolding.* Doing so is one of the ways you will ensure that you will walk the path of your destiny, your true path."

"I read a story about you in the paper a little while ago," I said. "It's incredible what you're doing to help make the world a better place."

"Yes, I read that article," Julian replied with a grin. "I actually have it with me somewhere. I am an idealist and it makes me feel so happy when I read that piece because I am reminded that I am making a difference. I measure my life not by decades but by deeds. I've learned that lasting happiness comes by giving, not getting. The Chinese say it so well: 'A little fragrance always clings to the hand that gives roses.' And yet we all too often forget that. In business, for example, we fail to act in win-win ways. We buy into the false assumption that someone has to lose for us to win. We guard our territories and refuse to operate from a frame of reference that sees the value in helping all those around us succeed. There's no truth in that. As a matter of fact, the best way to lead the field in business is to devote yourself to adding more value to your clients and customers than they have any right to expect. The true leaders in business understand who puts food on their tables and, therefore, treat their customers like royalty. They serve, cherish and love their customers. Love is an incredibly powerful business tool, you know?"

"I've never thought of it that way."

"Well, it's true, my friend. *And before anyone will lend you a hand, you must touch their heart.* Be like the sun: the sun gives all it can give. But in return, all of the flowers, the trees and the plants grow towards it. In your business life alone, by dedicating yourself to delighting and loving your clients, you will create an army of goodwill ambassadors who will run out into the world and tell everyone they know about what you do and who you are. Even when it comes to your so-called competition, try to do whatever you can to help them. Forge alliances with them. Develop friendships with them. Business is all about relationships. Help them get what they want and the ancient law of reciprocity will kick in—they'll begin to help you get what you want. Giving begins the receiving process."

"Very nice point," I agreed, sensing the power of this man's words.

"So, as I say, the bit about the difference I'm making in that article makes me feel good about myself since it reminds me I'm blessing lives, in my own small way. But I don't take all the recognition I'm getting too seriously. *No one takes you seriously when you take yourself too seriously, you know.*"

I smiled on hearing that line. This guy was good.

"I can't believe they're calling me a sage," he continued, lifting a speck of banana off his pristine robe. "What do I know about that kind of thing? I'm just an ordinary man who has, with the help of some very powerful teachers, discovered a philosophy that will lead anyone who chooses to adopt it to a beautiful life. Every human being needs to carve out the time to articulate a philosophy for his or her life—it's one of the most important things a person can do. Every person, to live truly and greatly, must define how he wants to live and what his brightest life will look like. We all need to have a statement on a piece of paper that we can revisit every morning while the rest of the world is asleep that will serve as a moral compass to direct the choices of our day. This will serve as an anchor to lock us into our best moves. Without such a statement of philosophy, you will live your life by accident, reacting to whatever pops up within your days. Living like that is a recipe for disaster— you're just begging for trouble when you live like that. Makes me think of a saying: 'If you don't know where you're going, any road will get you there.'"

"So I need to take some time to think about what I want my life to stand for?"

"Absolutely, Dar. This is one of the *musts* of life. Successful and fulfilled people make the time to think, plan and reflect. They are awake to their lives because they know that each day is an incredibly precious gift. If you don't believe that, walk into a hospital on the way home and talk to someone in the cancer ward. Ask them what they would give for an extra day of life."

What Julian said shot through me. I had taken so much of life for granted. I had never viewed each day above ground as a gift and an opportunity to create something great or make a difference.

"Most people spend more time planning their summer vacations than they do planning their lives. What a shame. Be thoughtful about your life. Ask yourself: 'How am I meant to live?' Question what you are meant to do, what things you will no longer tolerate in your life and what standards of excellence you will hold yourself to, on a go-forward basis. Living life without a devotion to excellence dishonors the priceless gifts and talents that have been given to you."

Julian continued, taking a few steps as he spoke and raising his hands into the air for effect. "Without a philosophy that reflects *your* truth in terms of how you want to live and what you aim to be, how can you make choices that are right for you? Without a philosophy, you will live your life according to other people's wishes. You'll be like those lemmings, following the crowd as they walk off the cliff to their deaths. *Without a philosophy, you just might find yourself on your deathbed and wonder 'what if my whole life was a lie?'"*

"That explains the writing on the card. The line about 'Stop living your life as a lie.' I assume you were the one who left that for me, Julian?"

"Of course. What fun is life without a hint of mystery? What joy is life without a little adventure? I was trying to inject some wonder into your life. This path you are interested in walking is not for the faint of heart, my friend. It requires great courage. You must confront your fears and then move through them. It will not be easy but it will lead you to the place that the deepest part of you is hungering to know. Anyway, as I was saying before, I can't believe people are calling me a guru. I'm just a student of life who has some pretty powerful insights to share. Think of me more as a guide. I drop into people's lives to guide them in the right direction. I look for people who have a *willingness* to make some big changes in their lives because they know, deep within, that there is so much more to life than what they are currently experiencing. Makes me think of what Rumi once said: 'Whoever enters The Way without a guide will take a hundred years to travel a two-day journey.'"

I chuckled, appreciating the depth of wisdom being shared. This *must* have been Julian Mantle. Who else could share what he was sharing? I relaxed even more, releasing the last bit of uncertainty about this unusual man's identity.

"Maybe a better way to look at what I do is to consider me a life coach. I coach people on becoming their highest selves and help them play their biggest games as human beings. I help people discover their destiny and live their dreams. *It's hard to believe that we live in a world where most people are more concerned with following the crowd and doing what everyone else is doing than living their dreams.* I'll tell you something I pray you never will forget: *One of the greatest regrets a person can ever have is getting to the end of their lives and realizing they did not do their dreams.* Getting to the end or even the middle of your life and waking up one day to the understanding that you did not dare, that you did not reach for the stars, that you did not realize even one-tenth of your potential will break your heart. Trust me on this one—I see it all the time. At the end of our lives, what fills our hearts with regret are not all the risks we took. Instead, what causes us to feel immense sadness is thinking about all the risks we *didn't* take, all the opportunities we did not seize, all the things we did not do. Do not live your life as a timid soul, my friend. Get into the arena, forget about the critics and play big with the gifts of your days. Life is short and the years will slip away very quickly, like grains of sand passing through your fingers on a hot day at the beach. You were meant to shine and let your talents see the light of day. *There is but one failure in life and that is the failure to try.* The greatest failure in life is the unwillingness to play your highest game and walk towards the places that frighten you."

"I agree, Julian. I completely agree. I regret so much of the way I've lived up until now."

"Be gentle with yourself. We grow from our mistakes. What's that expression—good judgment comes from experience, experience comes from making mistakes and mistakes come from bad judgment." I'd rather be willing to experiment with life and make a few mistakes than forego growth by refusing to step out of the confines of my comfort zone. So you made some mistakes. Forgive yourself and move on. *The past is a grave and it makes no sense to spend your life living in a grave. Every ending represents a new beginning. Or to put it another way, you cannot move forward in life if you're stuck looking in the rearview mirror.* As Cicero noted: 'The souls of wise people look to the future state of their existence; all of their thoughts are concentrated towards eternity.' The key is to *learn* from your mistakes and build a foundation of wisdom. Blend self-responsibility with self-forgiveness. The key is also to keep running towards rather than away from your fears because on the other side of your greatest fears lives your greatest life. If you do not keep running towards your fear wall, you will never—ever—discover personal freedom. Freedom lives on the other side of your fears. How often do you think most people are frightened?"

"I have no idea," I replied honestly. "Maybe once every few months."

"If you do not feel some fear on a *daily* basis, you are living life within a safe harbor and clinging to the shore. Do you know the story of how Columbus came to the New World?" Julian asked warmly.

"No, I don't, Julian. I used to read a lot of history but I have no idea what the answer to your question is."

"He went perpendicular," said Julian as he brought his bronzed hands together to form a "T."

"What do you mean by that?"

"Before Columbus, all previous adventurers sailed close to the shore, within sight of land. That was the accepted way to sail. Columbus dared to be different. He refused to do what all others had done. He took a risk: he sailed perpendicular to the shore—straight out to sea. And because he let go of the known and had the bravery to sail out into the unknown, he became one of our greatest heroes. You see, my friend, heroes are revolutionaries. All progress of humankind has been made by people who refused to think, feel and act like everyone else. John F. Kennedy stating he would work hard to put a man on the moon was the talk of a revolutionary, one who refused to follow the crowd and play small. Mahatma Gandhi's dream of freeing a nation was the fantasy of a revolutionary who refused to let his fears run him. Mother Teresa's goal of ridding Calcutta of the shackles of poverty was the ideal of a revolutionary who refused to listen to the shouts of the naysayers telling her it could not and should not be done. George Bernard Shaw said it so very well: 'The reasonable man adapts himself to the world; the unreasonable one tries to adapt the world to himself. Therefore, all progress depends on the unreasonable man.' That's such an important point of wisdom. All progress comes from unreasonable people, people who follow their hearts and the instructions of their consciences rather than the commands of the crowd. All progress has come from risk-takers and men and women who were willing to visit the places that scared them."

"That is a great point, Julian," I agreed. "All human progress, all of the advancements in the world—ranging from the discovery of fire to the creation of the personal computer—have come about by people who had the courage not to listen to the crowd but do what they felt was right, regardless of the fact it provoked uncertainty and fear within them."

"To take risks is to provoke fear, amigo. But to take risks is to be most alive. I deeply feel that we are most alive when we are taking risks, being bold and visiting the unknown spaces of our lives. *'Big risks, big life. Small risks, small life,'* is the way I view it. If you want to live greatly, you must also be willing to risk greatly. To get to the pearls, the diver needs to be willing to go deep and visit the places that the timid souls would never visit."

"Good example."

"When you ask for something you've never asked for from someone and your heart starts beating rapidly, that's when you are truly alive. When you want to say something to someone but the very thought of doing so sends butterflies through your stomach, that's when you are most alive. When you do something that you've never done before but follow through on it because you know in your heart it's something that will make your life richer and better, that's when you are most alive. Papa Wallenda, the great high-wire walker, said it so well when he observed: 'Life is on the wire. The rest is just waiting.'"

Julian continued with a level of enthusiasm that is rare in our world today. "So see me as your life coach. All smart businesspeople have coaches to help them get where they want to go. Every elite athlete has a coach to help them play at their best. Well, think of yourself as an elite performer on the playing field of life—you need a coach to guide, inspire and champion you as you evolve into who you are destined to become. I knew you'd be here at the seminar tonight. That guy was pretty good out there—I really liked what he had to say. I hope I didn't frighten you by the way I drew you to me."

"Oh no, Julian, you didn't," I lied.

Julian continued. "It's just that the people I work with must be people willing to take some risks. At each step along the journey of our lives, we have choice. We can confront the things that we are resisting, and in doing so grow as human beings. Or we can choose not to stretch ourselves and, in doing so, remain stagnant and small. In other words, our choices either free us or they limit us. So I placed a few little challenges in your way to see how you'd respond. And you did great."

"Well, Julian—and I hope you don't mind me calling you Julian . . ."

"Of course not, Dar. We'll be getting to know each other quite well over the coming weeks. Let's do away with any formality," replied Julian as he sipped from a bottle of Evian water.

"I'd love to have you as my life coach. Actually, I'm very honored that you would choose me as your next project. You're right. I have a great sense that I am ready to discover my destiny and live my true life. Something miraculous happened to me yesterday that opened up that awareness within me. I can't really get into it right now, but let me simply say that I'm beginning to appreciate what a treasure this gift of life is. I'm also starting to realize that each of us has far more potential for greatness than most of us can fathom."

"Very true," Julian affirmed.

I continued. "Julian, let me ask you a basic question that I think a lot of people are wondering about: how does one actually go about discovering his destiny?"

Julian ran a hand along the embroidery on the front of his robe. He closed his eyes, as if he was seeking guidance from a higher source. After a long silence, he spoke.

*"No one discovers their destiny, Dar. Your destiny will discover you—it will find you, provided you have done the preparation and inner work required to seize the opportunity when it presents itself.* Carlos Castaneda said it so well: 'All of us, whether or not we are warriors, have a cubic centimeter of chance that pops out in front of our eyes from time to time. The difference between the average person and a warrior is that the warrior is aware of this and stays alert, deliberately waiting, so that when this cubic centimeter of chance pops out, it is picked up.'"

"Neat."

"Here's the key. Stop worrying about finding your destiny. Spend your time getting to know *yourself.* Tear down the façade you show to the world and do the deep inner work on yourself needed to know who you really are. Focus on rebuilding your self-relationship. Get to know your deepest and truest values. Get to know your preferences and priorities—not those that others have taught you are the most important but those that *you* feel to be of the highest value. Get to know what genuinely makes you feel happy. Bring the subconscious patterns and ways of reacting to things out into the light of your awareness, so they can be healed. Get to know your fears and how you came to make them your own. As you come to know who you are, you can then claim your destiny as it draws closer to you. As you get to know who you truly are and what you are really all about, you will be able to seize that 'cubic centimeter of chance' when it pops out in front of you. And trust me, it will."

"Okay. Makes perfect sense. I'm open to doing all this 'inner work,' as you call it—even getting to know my darkest fears."

"Someone gave you your fears, you know? Someone taught them to you."

"Really?"

"Of course. At the moment of your birth, you were truly fearless. At the moment of your birth, you were pure perfection. Henri Amiel once wrote that 'Childhood is blessed by heaven because it brings a piece of paradise into the cruelties of life. All these thousands of everyday births are fresh additions of innocence and purity which fight against our spoiled nature.'"

"So true, Julian. Children do come to us more highly evolved than adults to teach us the lessons we need to learn. I know I've forgotten that lesson many times. In so many ways, children are the teachers. They know so much more than we allow them credit for."

"Exactly, amigo. As infants, we really are perfect. We are still connected to the force that created the world. But as we begin to age, we adopt fears from the world around us. We become 'spoiled.' We do this because we want to fit in and be like everyone else. We want our parents to love and adore us. So we model them and take on their fears, limiting beliefs and false assumptions so we can be more like them. It's all done because we crave to be loved. *Who you are in this moment is not who you truly are. Rather, it's someone you've become as a result of being in this world.* To clear all those fears that you have *assumed* from the world around you, you will need to go back and explore the source of all your fears. Then you'll have to work through them until they are no longer a part of your psyche. To know yourself so that your destiny will come calling, you must also pay more attention to your life and reflect on the lessons that need to be learned. You must be strict with yourself and examine your story."

"My story?"

"Every one of us creates a story about his own life, even if he only tells it to himself. For some, the story is all about being a victim. They are the way they are because of their childhoods or because of where they grew up or because of the bad things that have happened to them. So many people in the world today are professional victims."

"Why?"

"Because playing the victim is easy. You do not have to assume any responsibility for the way your life looks. You can blame everyone else for what's not working in your life, never having to look at yourself and make the changes required. *But when you play victim, you assign away your power to that which you allege is victimizing you. It's a very impotent way to live.*"

"So true," I replied, nodding my head in agreement.

"The story that people create may be that they are too old to chase their dreams or not attractive enough to find the mate they desire or not smart enough to do what they wish to do. It goes on and on. My point is really this: *The best move you can make is to work on your self-relationship.*"

"Just like you did in the Himalayas," I interjected.

"Just as I did in the Himalayas," Julian echoed. "Most people have lost the connection with themselves. They have forgotten who they truly are. That makes me so sad. Every single one of us has greatness written into our DNA. Our lives were meant to be joy-filled, exciting and rich with love, peace and beauty. Happiness is our birthright. But we get in our own way. We have fallen into the trap of mediocrity. We believe that we are not meant for miracles. We play small for fear that, should we step out into our higher possibilities, we will get hurt or people will not love us or our lives will not work."

"So true."

Julian continued enthusiastically. "We buy into the lie that only money will bring us happiness and so we sell our souls. We just don't know who we are anymore and what we were meant to become. We've unconsciously traded in the authentic power we are born with for the external power that comes from being in the world. We really have forgotten who we truly are. And if you do not know who you are and what it is you truly want to be, then how can you recognize and seize your destiny when it presents itself to you? *Know yourself and, I promise you, your destiny will find you.*"

Julian paused. "Okay, time to wrap up our first coaching session, Dar. It's getting late and I'm sure you've had enough excitement for one night."

Julian then put one of his muscular arms around my shoulders as we left the dressing room and walked down the hallway. Just being next to Julian brought me to peace.

"And all I ask is that you trust me. If you are willing, I will take you to a place you never dreamed of being. Frederick Faust said it well when he noted: 'There is a giant asleep within every person. When that giant awakes, miracles happen.' I will share the secrets that I learned high up in those mountains with you. I will show you all you need to know to

taste the deliciousness that life can be. Just 'let (
length of the reins' for once in your life, my friend."

"What do you mean by that?"

"Well, it's a phrase I love. It speaks to the need for each and every one of us to walk into our fears, if we want to live big and gorgeous lives. It comes from something Mary Cholmondeley once wrote. Here, take this. It'll be helpful."

Julian handed me a slip of paper from the pocket of his robe. It looked crumpled from much use. It read simply:

*Every year I live I am more convinced that the waste of life lies in the love we have not given, the powers we have not used, the selfish prudence that will risk nothing, and which, shirking pain, missed happiness as well. No one ever yet was poorer in the long run having once in a lifetime 'let out all the length of the reins.'*

"Amazing quote, Julian. Please know that I'm willing to do whatever you advise me to do," I replied quickly, recognizing the giant opportunity that Julian's life coaching invitation presented. I'd been hearing a lot about the value of having a life coach from many of my friends who also ran businesses, and I felt blessed that Julian had entered my life at this point in time. "How long will my transformation take?"

*"Personal transformation is not a race, Dar. Actually, sometimes the harder you try to change, the longer it takes.* So many people treat self-discovery like an extreme sport—rushing to get all their healing at a frenetic pace. They read book after book. They visit guide after guide and attend seminar

after seminar. They want to know the answers to the big questions they are struggling with. But someone who cannot sit in the mystery of their lives and enjoy the process of personal growth is a person in fear."

"Really?" I asked, surprised to hear this. One of the dominant values of our society is "faster is better" and to hear Julian reject this notion only heightened the mystique that surrounded him and his untraditional philosophy.

"Trust that your timing is not necessarily nature's timing. Relax into the process. You are not meant to know all the answers, at least not right now. When you are ready for a piece of learning and a specific lesson, it will come. What fun would it be if you knew all the plot twists of a movie half-way into it? *Your life is like a thriller, my friend—half the fun is not knowing what's going to happen. Life is so fluid. Everything's always changing. The way you think it's going to unfold is not the way it's going to unfold. That's the fun of the whole exercise. That's also the gift.*"

"What do you mean?"

"Part of the purpose of life is to learn to simply *accept* that it's all a mystery. Part of what your whole journey is about is to *learn to let go* of all your fears about it not working out the way you want it to work out. Life will never work out the way you expect it to. Once you know that you can begin to relax and enjoy the adventure of it all. Just look back on the way your life has unfolded to date. Has it turned out as you planned it would?"

"I've often thought, over the past few months, that I never imagined it would look like this."

"Right. Everybody's life is like that. And if you reflect on my question longer and dig deeper, I predict that you will discover that while you may not have expected some of the lows, the same could be said for the high points of your life."

"Yeah, that's completely true, Julian. I'm going through a really hard time right now but, to be honest, I'll admit that I never dreamed I would have enjoyed all the successes I've had along the way. Totally unexpected how wonderful many things have turned out."

"Exactly. So the lesson really is that no one can control life or understand its grand design. But, trust me, there is a perfection to it. Even what you are now experiencing you will, over the passage of time, come to see as a beautiful blessing that has added enormous value and richness to your life."

"Seriously?"

"Seriously," said Julian.

He added: "Too many people can't handle the notion that their plans and goals will not pan out as they anticipate. That kind of thinking reflects a control issue on their part. And behind their need to control is often fear. These people do not trust in nature's ways. Such people have little faith in the love the source of all creation has for them. Yes, make plans and set goals. Work hard and go for what you desire. That's part of being a responsible person—it is true that setting intentions does make many of them to come to life. *But hold on to your plans and goals with a very loose grip*. Often, the universe will send you a treasure in an unexpected package. If you are so busy holding on to—and hunting down—what you think is best for you, you may miss what's *truly* best for you."

"I have never heard anything like this. Those sages in India must have been pretty amazing people."

"That's an understatement, my friend. So, back to what I was sharing," said Julian, maintaining a laserlike focus on the point he wanted me to grasp, "let go of your need to control the path of your destiny. Because, no matter how hard you try, you just can't. Sure, you can make wise choices and your choices will have an impact. But ultimately, you are not in control. We are so arrogant as human beings. We think that we are more intelligent than the universe. This universe that created the sunsets and the rainbows. This universe that created the stars and the moon. We think that we know more about what's in our best interests than the source that created all that exists. It's even funny when you think about it. We of so little faith."

"It *is* all our fear, I'm beginning to appreciate."

"Correct," replied Julian. "Fear is the number one factor that causes people to live small, inauthentic lives. To go back to your original question about how long transformation takes, I want to repeat that personal growth is not a big race to the finish line. Instead, it's a very *organic* process. You must allow time for the lessons I will reveal to you to become integrated within the depths of your being. When you are ready to receive a certain lesson, you will receive a perfect experience or person who will represent an opportunity for you to learn that lesson. And once you get the lesson, time must elapse so you can integrate it. There's no hurry. It's all a lovely journey. Trust that where you are, at any given point, is precisely where you are meant to be."

"Okay, I'll loosen up a little more. I see that it's not a race. I'll let my transformation unfold 'organically,' as you say, Julian," I remarked.

Julian led me down the long hallway that would bring us back to the auditorium. Seeing an empty soda can that someone had thrown on the cement floor, he reached down and picked it up. "Every small act counts," he said. I wasn't quite sure what he meant by this comment but I remained silent.

"Over the coming weeks and months, I will share a seven-stage process that will help you reclaim the perfection you knew as a newborn child. This process will awaken the highest and best within you. But you must be patient. If you follow it to its absolute conclusion, you will taste enlightenment as a human being."

"Enlightenment? Wow!" I said, sensing the joy that was awaiting me.

"You must commit to this journey, Dar. You must be willing to do the inner work required to move through The 7 Stages of Self-Awakening and bravely walk the path I will reveal to you. Please know that, at every step of the way, you will have a choice—human beings always have choice in the way their destinies unfold. You can resist the growth that I'm going to encourage you to take or you can embrace it. And if you keep choosing to grow and walk in the direction of your fears, you will move to higher and higher stages of personal freedom and individual greatness. You will be able to discover what life's really all about. You will begin to know the universal truths and natural laws that govern the operation of the world. Once you know these, you can keep choosing to align yourself with them. And when you align yourself with the natural laws that run the world, your life *automatically* works. You begin to discover the truth. You begin to know who you truly are. You begin to access your personal brilliance and the limitless possibilities that lie at the essence of your life. That's when your life becomes magic."

"Will this cost anything, Julian?" I asked, as we entered the auditorium where the motivational speaker had spoken earlier in the evening. "I've heard personal coaching can be very expensive."

"Of course not. My services are free—just keep me well supplied with bananas," Julian said with a grin. "Seriously, I'm on a crusade to help people realize what they're truly made of. It is my highest joy to help a person in need of my knowledge. *Selfless service is the rent I pay for living on this wonderful planet.* I want people to know what it means to be a fully functioning, self-awakened human being. It hurts me to see the shape the world is in," observed Julian as he stopped walking. He was silent for a moment and perfectly still but for the tears that began to well up in his eyes.

"It is a place where people have forgotten how to dream. I want to help people dream again. Wouldn't it be incredible if the human race could come together as a band of dreamers? Imagine what our world would look like. Imagine the legacy we could leave behind for our children! I want to help people trust again. I want to help people live again. And I mean *truly* live. I want to show people how to *love* again. So, my friend, it is my *duty* to help you. It will be a joy to be of service to you. I'm a servant leader in the truest sense of the word, if you don't mind my saying so. Giving to others provides me with great happiness. That is more than enough of a reward," Julian said.

"I'm grateful, Julian," I said, expressing my heartfelt appreciation for this man who was so interested in helping me.

"The word 'duty' is often viewed negatively in our culture.

Many people don't like the idea of it, feeling that duty would restrict them and hinder them from living in the moment. To me, the word 'duty' represents freedom and happiness. The great Indian poet Rabindranath Tagore said it far more elegantly than I ever could: 'I slept and dreamt life was Joy, and then I awoke and realized life was Duty. And then I went to work—and lo and behold, I discovered that Duty can be Joy.' My destiny is to serve. And doing what I am meant to do—performing the work that I have been placed on the planet to perform—is sheer joy and absolute bliss for me. Woodrow Wilson spoke truth when he observed: *'You are here not merely to make a living. You are here in order to enable the world to live more amply, with greater vision, with a finer spirit of hope and achievement. You are here to enrich the world, and you impoverish yourself if you forget that errand.'*"

"Okay, Julian," I replied. "I promise you that I will be a great student. I'll listen to your wisdom. I commit to making the changes that you will suggest. Thank you for finding me. Thank you so much. I have a sense that my life will never be the same after tonight."

"You're right about that, my friend. Meet me at The Q Hotel tomorrow morning. We will begin our first full lesson then."

"That's one of my hotels," I laughed.

"I know," said Julian, beaming. "I'm staying there. Like I said, there's nothing wrong with living a materially beautiful life. Just don't make it what you're all about."

"It's great to know that. Awakening my best self wouldn't be so fun if I had to give up everything I've worked so hard for. Some of these things, like my sailboat, make me so happy. I love being out on the water on a perfect summer day. For a while there, I thought you were going to tell me that the only way I could find enlightenment is to sell everything I own and go live on a mountaintop in isolation."

"I believe that in many ways that would be a cop-out, actually. Anyone can find a certain degree of peace by divorcing themselves from the world and spending their lives in solitude. No one and nothing can press your buttons when you are all alone. I'll never forget reading about a monk who had spent seven years in solitude, living in one of the temples of Tibet. He would often go for months in silence, stilling his mind and ridding it of impurities. A time came when he felt he had reached the state of enlightenment. So do you know what he did?"

"Tell me."

"He returned to New York City. On the day of his return, he went out to do some shopping in that glorious metropolis. Within minutes, he was overcome by stress. The honking horns, the swelling crowds and the frenetic pace frightened him. Hardly the response of an enlightened being. Now, I'm not saying that silence and solitude are *not* important in reconnecting with your highest self. Kahlil Gibran, the brilliant philosopher, once wrote: 'There is something greater and purer than what the mouth utters. Silence illuminates our souls, whispers to our hearts, and brings them together. Silence separates us from ourselves, makes us sail the firmament of spirit, and brings us closer to heaven.'"

"Beautiful words," I said, luxuriating in the profound quote Julian had just shared.

"They are. So silence and solitude are essential for you to take part in all the possibilities that your life is meant to offer. But what really takes courage and strength of character is to find enlightenment right here in the middle of the city. What really takes wisdom is to find inner peace right where you are."

"What about the monks you met? I wonder how they would have reacted in New York City?" I wondered aloud.

"These monks are known as the Sages of Sivana. Few people have ever been able to find them, as they are extremely reclusive and reside in a particularly remote part of the Himalayas. And you should know that these monks are *genuinely* enlightened beings. Put them *anywhere* in the world and place them in *any* situation and I promise you they will remain perfectly at ease, deeply at peace. These sages were nothing less than magical people. I know I'll never meet human beings like them again," said Julian as he glanced towards the floor. I guessed he was missing them.

"What time do you want to meet at The Q in the morning?" I asked gently.

"Five A.M."

"You're kidding."

"Would I kid you about something like that, amigo?" asked Julian with a wink, perking up. "If you want the wisdom of a monk you need to play like one. The sages believed that the hours of the very early part of the morning have an almost mystical quality that offer an excellent space for learning and deepening."

And with that statement of belief, Julian reached over and gave me a quick hug and strode down the hallway, robe swaying from side to side. I remained there, standing in silence for several minutes. I literally did not move. I could not believe my good fortune. Just when I thought I would never find the answers I had been seeking, a genuine Master had appeared in my life.

Making my way out of the auditorium, I saw that someone had dropped a leather wallet on the floor. I picked it up, with the intention of giving it to a security guard or late-night supervisor. My curiosity got the better of me and I couldn't help opening it up to check the contents. There was no money and no credit cards or other pieces of identification inside it. In fact, the wallet was empty except for one thing: within the billfold was something that surprised me. It was a copy of the article that our local newspaper had written on Julian and his adventures. I removed it and stared at it. Julian had obviously left this for me. The last two sentences of the article had been underlined in red. They read: "Julian Mantle—The Monk Who Sold His Ferrari—believes in the power of the human spirit to be a force for good in the world. He appears to have discovered the truths upon which every glorious life has been built and maybe, if you are very lucky, you will be his next student."

I folded the paper and placed it in my shirt pocket—the one next to my heart.

# CHAPTER 3

# The Seeker Learns the Power of a Calling and About the Hidden Meaning of Destiny

*Just imagine that the purpose of life is your happiness only—then life becomes a cruel and senseless thing. You have to embrace the wisdom of humanity. Your intellect and your heart tell you that the meaning of life is to serve the force that sent you into the world. Then life becomes a joy.*

—Leo Tolstoy

I tossed and turned during that short night of sleep, and had some of the strangest dreams I'd ever had. I dreamt I was running through the streets naked. I had another dream in which I was locked in my car as it ran off a bridge and into the sea. And I had yet another dream in which I possessed the happy ability to fly. Each of these dreams, I guessed, had some significance for what I was going through. "Dreams are the language of the soul," I'd read somewhere.

Running through the streets naked was probably about my heart's longing for me to be more vulnerable and taking off the façade—the public mask—I'd worn all my life in an effort to fit in and be like everyone else. The dream was likely about being more authentic, but also about the fear of being open. Being locked in the sinking car probably spoke to the fears that had started coming up after Julian left me last night. I began to doubt some of the things he told me. Could I really transform my life? Would my destiny really unfold if I simply went within and got to know myself? Was it true that most people had resigned themselves to lives of mediocrity and missed out on the dazzling existence that was meant for them? And what about Julian's 7 Stages of Self-Awakening? While I did trust Julian, and his intellectual brilliance was beyond challenge, some of what he had shared with me seemed so very mystical.

And the dream about flying, well, my gut told me that had something to do with the deepest part of me—my soul—craving to rise to my highest potential. I thought of the words that came to me in the motel room, only two days before: *Life is a treasure and you are so much more than you know.* Thinking over my dreams in the early-morning darkness, I began to feel more and more sure that, with Julian as my wise and caring coach, my life couldn't help but soar.

The Q Hotel was one of my favorite properties in our boutique hotel portfolio. It was stylish and very popular among the fashionistas and the jet-set. I had woken up at 4:30 A.M. with much difficulty but I didn't want to be late for my meeting with Julian. I knew that he was a punctual man who valued promise-keeping. My dad had told me so.

As I drove up to The Q, with its chic, minimalist look, I couldn't help noticing the stunning car parked right out front. It was a classic Ferrari. Red, gleaming—in mint condition. I couldn't take my eyes off it. It immediately brought back memories of my childhood when my father and I used to drive by Julian's sprawling mansion and stare at his car.

I really missed my dad. He was a great man. He passed away a number of years ago, and I still feel sadness when I think about it. I miss him every day. I also miss my kids a lot. Sure, I see them every week but they are a part of my heart and I wish they could be with me all the time. Anyway, as I say, the Ferrari brought back a flood of memories, really good ones.

As I parked my car behind the Ferrari, the new bellman, Jake, hurried over to greet me.

"Good morning, Mr. Sandersen, and welcome to The Q," he said with a laugh. "It's really great to see you, Boss."

"Great to see you too, Jake," I replied sincerely. "Whose baby is this?" I asked, pointing to the car.

"I'm not sure. All I know is that we have a monk staying in the hotel this week. Everyone's talking about him. He drove up in it at about four o'clock this morning, just after I started my shift. The guy really knows how to drive a Ferrari—you should have seen him racing up the street! The guy's pretty cool, if you don't mind my saying so—he even tipped me a twenty."

The great Julian Mantle, always full of surprises. I knew he had few possessions—the newspaper article confirmed this. It said that he wasn't interested in going back to his old lifestyle. But I knew Julian still enjoyed *all* aspects of living, this was clear. He made no apologies for his love of life's luxuries and his taste for the best. It was more a case of these sorts of things no longer sitting atop his list of life's priorities. While he enjoyed these things for the pleasures they offered, he had absolutely no requirement for them.

I had no idea where Julian got the Ferrari from and did not know how he had enough money to stay at The Q. *I just trusted that everything was in perfect order in the universe.* I shook Jake's hand and entered the lobby. Maria, the beautiful Italian concierge, greeted me. "Mr. Mantle is waiting for you up in his room, Mr. Sandersen. I wish you a wonderful morning."

"Which room's he in, Maria?"

"We gave him the Lotus Loft."

"That's one of the most expensive rooms in the hotel!" I said with surprise.

"Well, he came in here and asked for a room. He said it didn't matter which room we gave him, he would be comfortable with anything. And he was so polite and friendly. So we gave him our favorite room in the hotel. I just love the Lotus Loft—it's not the biggest but it has the best energy, as far as I'm concerned."

I just shook my head and smiled. I walked towards the elevators and rode one up to Julian's floor. As I walked down the hallway to Julian's room, I could hear someone singing along to some recorded music. It wasn't loud enough to wake any of our sleeping guests, but it was noticeable. As I drew closer to my destination, I realized the rock star wannabe was (of course) none other than the great Julian Mantle.

As soon as I knocked on the door, it opened . . . to an amazing sight: Julian was standing there with a huge smile, wearing nothing more than a pair of crisp white boxer shorts. His body was lithe and tanned, striations from his taut muscles peeked out from the skin. I had seldom seen anyone in such outstanding physical condition and certainly not a man who was about the same age as my father would have been, had he still been alive. Julian's hair was stylishly swept back and he looked peaceful but energetic. In his hand he held a glass of orange juice.

"Good morning, amigo, c'mon in," he said with great gusto. "I'm just listening to some music. It's Dave Matthews—the song's called 'Gravedigger.' I love it. To me, it speaks to the importance of living fully while we have the chance to do so. Living full out. Enjoying every moment, even the less than ideal ones. Because soon life will be over. Before we know it, we'll be six feet under and all those simple pleasures we took for granted, like feeling raindrops on our faces or watching our children laugh or seeing the sun come up, will be things of the past. I'll tell you something, Dar: generally the things that we value most when we are in our twenties, thirties and forties become the things we value least at the end of our lives. And all those things that so many among us currently value least, like deep human connections, random acts of kindness, being in superb physical condition, devoting ourselves to excellence in our work, creating a legacy and carving out time each day to work on ourselves so that the best within us shines, will—in the end—reveal themselves to be most valuable. *On our deathbeds, no one wishes they had more money in their bank accounts or a bigger car sitting in the driveway. Instead, as we take our last few breaths, we wish that we had lived a life that was courageous, authentic and highly loving.*"

"So true. And yet we spend the best years of our lives chasing things like fame and fortune."

"Right. We do so because we are taught by those around us that these are the values that matter. But we have a choice: we can buy into the values of the crowd or we can dare to be true to ourselves and live life on the terms that feel right to us, at our most deep and true level. Again, there's nothing wrong with money. It's actually a wonderful thing that brings much happiness and does much good if properly handled. Making money is great and it *should* be one of your priorities if you desire to live a beautiful life."

"It's just that the pursuit of money should not be my highest priority."

"Exactly. Never make the mistake of placing it above your commitments to serve the force that sent you here, to make a difference while you walk the planet, to love your family and to reclaim your biggest self. Remember that there are many forms of wealth, financial wealth being only one of them. One who has rich relationships and a loving community around her is, in my mind, wealthy. One who has a life of adventure, excitement and continuous learning has wealth of a different sort. And one who is spiritually connected to all of life and wakes up every morning feeling deeply at peace and aware of the truth must certainly be considered to be one who has accumulated yet another form of riches. The crowd—our tribe called society—has taught us that economic wealth is the only type of wealth we should chase. A lie. And please consider this essential fact about money: money is only a *byproduct*."

"A byproduct of what?"

"Of adding value and doing good for others. Focus on being

great at what you do. Dedicate yourself to offering others all you can to make their lives better. Be *truly* outstanding in every element of your professional and your personal life. The money will follow, this I guarantee you. You see, Dar, *money is the unintended yet inevitable byproduct of a life spent helping others get what they want. Money is nothing more than payment rendered by the universe in return for value you have added to others. As you sow, so shall you reap."*

"Uh, Julian," I interjected, "where are your robes? I know that last night you said we should strip away the formalities, but isn't this a little much? Nice boxers, though," I said with a chuckle. I knew I could be playful with Julian—he was a fun guy.

"My robes are being dry-cleaned, Dar. Quite the staff you have here—I'm impressed. They said they'd have them back in a few hours. So for now, I'm relaxing in my boxers. Just loving this music—music makes my soul sing. It's so important to me in my life. It makes me feel incredibly good. I couldn't imagine life without music."

A monk who loves Dave Matthews, chic hotels and good things. Pinch me. Julian polished off his glass of orange juice and then turned off the CD player. He looked at me apologetically. "I hope I didn't embarrass you by wearing these shorts to the door. I didn't give my attire a second thought. I was just having so much fun this morning. One of the things that I've developed as a result of meeting the Sages of Sivana in India is what I call 'a lust for life.' Everyone must do what they need to do to develop a lust for life. We all must make the time to get excited about the simple pleasures of life, the ones we cherished as children. For me, those pleasures are things like skipping stones across the water or making angels in the snow on a crisp winter's day. Or dancing to music as if you were completely alone. I get so caught up in the moment these days, I sometimes forget about some of the social graces that I used to worry about when I was a litigator. None of that kind of thing seems important to me anymore. Being fully engaged in the present—now that's so much of what life's all about. Nothing's more important to me than being here fully. *Life is lived in the now,* my friend. Like I said before, the past is a grave. Life is for the living. The wise among us get that. As the great writer and philosopher Paulo Coelho confirmed in his beautiful book *The Alchemist,* 'I'm interested only in the present. If you can concentrate only on the present, you'll be a happy man. You'll see that there is life in the desert, that there are stars in the heavens and that tribesmen fight because they are part of the human race. Life will be a party for you, a grand festival, because life is the moment we're living right now.'"

"Should I be writing all these lessons down, Julian?" I asked earnestly.

"No, not for now. Writing things down is an incredibly important practice for self-discovery. The monks I met up in the Himalayas taught me about the tremendous value of daily journaling. The discipline changed my life, Dar. Just as you get to know another person by having deep conversations with them, by journaling every morning you will come to know yourself through writing. I discovered what I wanted and what was holding me back from living my greatest life. My journal offered me a place to record my learning, an outlet to process through unfelt emotions that were blocking me and a vehicle to articulate the philosophy that I promised myself I would live by. But, though journaling can be wonderful for emotional clearing and healing, it is also a mind-centered activity. And for now, I want you to move away from your mind and closer to your heart. I want to guide you from your intellect into your feelings. You've lived your whole life in the mind and where has it brought you?"

"I'm still miserable," I replied in all honesty.

"Okay, so maybe, just maybe, there's an element or two that's missing," Julian offered in a kind tone. "My guess is that you need to open up your heart, my friend. And living in the moment happens in the heart, not the mind. Have you ever sat before a stunning sunset and found yourself thinking about work or about your schedule for that day or about some problem you were dealing with rather than paying attention to the perfection of the scene right in front of you?"

"Sure."

"Well, that happened because your mind was running the show. *The mind is an excellent servant but a tyrannical master.* The mind is a splendid *tool*, to be used for planning, patient reflection and learning from past mistakes so they will not be repeated, to use but a few examples. The mind will help you gain knowledge and receive education from life's teachings. But the mind must not run the show, as it does for most people. Balance living in the mind with operating from the heart, as I told you last night. It's that all-important harmony or partnership between head and heart. The heart wants you to take in every gift of that sunrise. The heart knows that life is lived in the present moment."

Julian fell silent. The Lotus Loft looked out over the entire city, an exquisite view. *Travel and Leisure* said this was one of the best hotel rooms in the world.

"Hey, what's with the car?" I asked, as I remembered the Ferrari downstairs. "I heard you drove it over here early this morning. Don't you sleep?"

"Sure I do. A good rest is essential for the body. I just don't sleep as much as most people do. Life is short and I don't waste my time. I could die tomorrow—who knows? So I live each day completely. Life's too much fun to miss out on. I have a calling to fulfill and a legacy to leave. I have been given some wonderful gifts and have a mission to pursue, one that I pray will help many people live richer lives. *Once you connect with some kind of higher purpose and main aim in your life, there will be a corresponding release of passion and energy into your life. The secret of generating extraordinary levels of passion in your life is to discover your larger purpose.* Once you find your calling, you get excited. And the greater excitement you will feel for this calling and for your life in general, the less you will need—or want—to sleep. Most people use sleep as a drug. They use sleep to distract them and pass the time. As people begin to live a life that is incongruent with their biggest lives and their highest possibilities, a well of pain begins to form within them. Most people are not conscious of this—it happens at the subconscious level—but that does not mean it's not there, affecting them in every moment, in every choice and at every plane. So many among us use sleep to avoid that pain."

"That's an interesting perspective, Julian. I've never considered that. I've always thought of pain as something more overt," I recognized.

Julian nodded, then continued. "But look at people who discovered a cause that they gave their lives over to, people such as Benjamin Franklin, Mahatma Gandhi, Martin Luther King Jr., Mother Teresa and Nelson Mandela. They connected with some kind of a crusade that they decided their lives would stand for. This engaged their hearts. This made them emotionally charged up about what they were doing. *And once you can develop some emotional engagement around a pursuit, rather than simply an intellectual one, the excitement flows and the energy explodes.* That's the big idea for you to think about at this point, my friend. Connect to a compelling cause with your heart, not your head. And then fasten your seatbelt because your life will soar."

"Do I have to leave the business world and my current job to find this cause that my life must stand for? The people you mention were freedom fighters and social activists. No offence, Julian, but those kinds of things just aren't *me*."

"Excellent point. Of course you can find your cause—your crusade—exactly where you are. No one has to leave a job to find something to engage their heart and excite them. Often, all that is required is that they see things differently. For example, you, as an owner of these hotels, can make a profound difference in many people's lives. Now that's something to get excited about."

"I can?"

"Sure. All the people who work for you spend more time at work than they do at home. They leave their families each morning and come in here to help you build your dream. Imagine that—they give you some of the best hours of the days of their lives. So in return for this gift, what if, through your efforts, you did whatever it took to create a workplace where it was safe to be human again. Imagine what it would do for your employees if being at work was a thing of joy for them and a place where they could grow, learn and let their natural creativity come out to play. What if you made it a priority to make their work fun and molded the culture into a place where noble values were the norm. You can create this kind of a culture at each of your wonderful hotels if you choose to do so. All it takes is time, effort and some innovation. I was in London recently and stayed at Ian Schrager's St. Martin's Lane. That hotel is the ideal example of a place where people are having fun, being innovative and loving their work. And, I must tell you, their passion was contagious. I loved my time there. Remember, *people love doing business with people who love doing business.*"

"Yes, that's true," I noted.

"Just imagine how energized you will feel knowing that you are creating a special place for human beings to work and do business. And if you make some shifts in perception, you can not only discover this cause by serving the people who work for you. You can also generate an enormous amount of excitement and emotional engagement when you think about what you can do for each customer who walks through your doors. Through your efforts and the efforts of your team, you can create beautiful memories. You can make them laugh and feel good. Many of them are on vacation and you can bring great joy to their lives by showing up at your best. Imagine waking up each morning and devoting yourself to creating 'unforgettable experiences' for your customers. Would this excite you?"

"Definitely. I'm feeling so inspired and excited even thinking about the opportunity. And the deeper I go on these kinds of commitments, the more I can see my excitement levels soaring. Now I get why you sleep less than most of us—you're connected and committed to a special purpose. And it's clear that your 'cause,' as you call it, fuels and energizes you."

"Yes, Dar. It gives me hope and gives me *so* much energy. *A cause to stand for, no matter if it's one about creating incredible experiences for the men and women who give you business or one that involves saving the world, unleashes energy.* Big idea to remember. When you connect to some main aim that taps into the highest and best you have to give, the greatest part of you feels you are spending your life in a worthy way. Your heart starts to open and pound, as never before. You see, my friend, the intellect—while it's useful in planning, reflecting and learning—is often limiting. The mental chatter that fills most people's minds is mostly about why we shouldn't do something and the adverse consequences of failure. The mind all too often keeps us small. *The heart and the emotions are the liberators. They cause us to step up to the plate and reach for greatness. They create excitement and passion and invite our biggest selves to come out to play.*"

"I definitely see the value of what you are sharing. My guess is that discovering a cause or crusade is also what keeps people going through tough times."

"Superb point!" exclaimed Julian. "My you are a wonderful student, Dar—one of the best yet." He walked over and inhaled the scent of a single rose that was standing in a simple, silver vase. "Leonardo da Vinci said it so well when he observed, 'Fix your course to a star and you can navigate any storm.' Once you know your main aim in life—this central mission of which I speak—it will serve as a North Star for you, guiding you through both good and bad times."

Julian paused and passed one of his bronzed hands through his hair. "Forgive me for going off on a bit of a tangent in reply to your question about why I sleep less but I know you realize that what I've just shared with you is extremely important for the creation of your best life. Find your cause, and then do your work with pride and love—love is such an incredible force for good. Do it with a devotion to excellence. The world will reward you in unimaginable ways."

"Pride, love and a devotion to excellence—love those terms."

"*Positive* pride is such an important element in the creation of a beautiful life. You know, Mahatma Gandhi once said: 'No matter how insignificant the thing you have to do, do it as well as you can, give as much of your care and attention as you would give to the thing you regard as most important. For it will be by those small things that you shall be judged.' Here's the sequence, Dar: when you devote yourself to excellence in *every* thing you do, from your role as a leader here at work to your role as a father in your personal life, you begin to feel a greater sense of positive pride about the way you are conducting your days. This in turn increases self-respect and confidence which, in turn, release greater energy and passion. That 'lust for life' I was telling you about earlier begins to kick in. You begin to feel good about yourself. People who feel good about themselves do great work and create great things. And this, in turn, just makes them raise their standards of excellence even higher. It's an upward spiral that takes people to ever-increasing places of joy, meaning and internal peace."

"Hearing this really inspires me, Julian," I said, as I sat down on the sleek designer sofa near the large window. "Now, let me ask you, do each of us have a *specific* calling that it is our duty to discover and then follow if we want to live authentic lives?"

"Big question, my friend. No one really knows the answer to that, do they? Many pretend they do though, if you read all those books out there in which the authors write as if they have a direct connection to the source of all creation. Unless you are enlightened, you can't know the answer—the best you can do is to discover a way of understanding how life works that feels right for you. I personally have come to believe that there is a very general pre-scripted plan for our lives that has been written in advance of our lives. Call it fate if you will. Having said that, I also believe that each and every one of us has an *incredible* amount of choice in the way our lives ultimately unfold and it is by our specific choices that our ultimate destinies are created. It's almost as though a rough design or sketch of our lives has been made for us by that wise architect in the sky and it falls to us to draw out the details. I need to say it again: we have tons of say in how our lives end up looking. We can have the lives we dream of, in so many ways. There's no doubt that as human beings, we cannot control all that happens to us—that's the fate part. Life runs along according to its own course. But what we do have enormous control over is the way we respond to what life sends our way. So that's the partnership: *do your best—the very best that you know how to do in every dimension of your life—and then let life do the rest. It's really a delicate balance between making it happen and letting it happen.* We really can make our own luck, a lot of the time, and good things generally happen to people who do good things. It's not as if life will happen according to a blueprint and the way you show up makes no difference. That's nonsense and a myth fostered by people afraid to assume personal responsibility over the conduct of their lives. But once you've done your absolute best, *let go and trust that whatever comes is perfectly suited for the growth you need to evolve into your best self.*"

"Which is really what you have been suggesting is the purpose of life, Julian, right?"

"Yes, I believe the purpose of life is growth and self-remembering. Growing into and remembering the brilliant creatures that we first were, the instant we were born—before we took on all the garbage of the world around us that soiled our perfection. Before we became spoiled and fell asleep to the truth about who we are and what beautiful and brave things we are destined to do."

"I'm still not quite sure about whether we have a *specific* calling or destiny, Julian. I know this is a complicated area and a big question, but it's important to me. Is there a specific job that I am meant to perform? Is there a specific woman—a soul mate—I am meant to find? Could you please elaborate a little on these points?"

"You're right—these are very challenging questions. Good for you for asking," said Julian, clearly pleased. He walked over to me and patted me on the back with a warm smile.

"First, let me suggest again that, in many ways, there are no answers to your questions. You are trying to understand that which is not understandable, at a human level, with our limited perception. But the fact that you're asking means you are going deep and thinking about a life philosophy that will fit you. While a part of me wants to say that these are simply life's mysteries, another part of me wants to tell you that I have a gut feeling about the answers you are seeking. And please know that the sages I met in India were enlightened souls who discovered so many of the truths that the average human being has not been able to access, so much of what I tell you comes from a very reliable source."

"I understand," I said, feeling slightly impatient to hear a series of little-known secrets that would change my understanding forever.

"Here's the way I believe it all works. Many possible paths to our best lives have been written for us. There are many doorways into the mansion of bliss. Just as there are many routes you can take to get home from work, there are many routes you can take to get to your biggest life, the life that has been meant for you—and getting there is a homecoming of sorts as well. There are many jobs you can take that will get you to your destiny. Similarly, there are many soul mates available to you, each offering different lessons, but all able to help you grow into and awaken your best self. Getting to your highest self and biggest life is the main purpose of life. Getting home to the place of brilliance, love and fearlessness you have forgotten is the reason for your existence. Now, it's up to you which route or path you take as you attempt to get to your authentic life. No one path is better than the other—they just look different. Taking one path might mean a longer trip, just like taking one particular route home may mean you need to travel a longer distance and face a few bumpier roads. Taking another path might be like taking an expressway to your destination, with a smooth ride and cloudless blue skies. It's up to you. It is, in large part, determined by the choices you make within the moments of your days. *You co-write the script that has been written for the story of your life, my friend.*"

"Okay, Julian, so now I need to ask: How does one go about taking those express routes to the place we are meant to be, according to this rough and general plan that you've mentioned has been set for our lives?"

"*Just do good and be good,*" came the direct reply. "This world of ours is run according to a series of immutable natural laws, laws created by the same force of nature that built the world and sent you here. You cannot play a game like soccer without knowing the rules. Well, life's like a game as well. And in order to play—and win—it's essential that you learn the rules. Live your life in alignment with them and your life will work. The universe wants you to win, did you know that? You just need to get out of your own way and figure out the rules to the game as quickly as you can. And learning the rules of the game takes some effort, deep thinking in silent places and a genuine willingness to be a philosopher."

"To be a philosopher?" I questioned.

"Sure. The definition of 'philosophy' is 'a love of wisdom.' Everyone, if they hope to walk the path of their destinies to their biggest lives, must develop an appreciation of wisdom and a hunger to understand what their life is all about. This world would be a much better place if we all began to view ourselves as philosophers, thoughtfully—and artfully—being in the process of sculpting more delightful and meaningful lives. So, back to these timeless natural laws, govern your daily actions by them and you will automatically take the expressway to your greatest life. Disregard them and you'll be taking the long way home."

"What are these natural laws anyway?" I asked, anxious to know more.

"They are the laws that have governed the operation of the world since it began. They include core principles such as 'always help others get what they want while you get what you want,' 'have impeccable integrity,' 'live in the present moment,' 'become the kindest person you know,' 'do your best and be excellent in all you do,' 'be true to yourself' and 'dream bravely.' Most of us know them but few of us live by them. It's like what Voltaire once said: 'Common sense is anything but common.'"

"That's true, Julian. These days, it's almost as though if something is not complex and sophisticated, we place little value on it. Yet, most truths really are simple, aren't they?"

"If it wasn't simple, it wouldn't be a truth," replied Julian sagely.

"Now you say 'Govern your actions by these natural laws and you will take the expressway to your greatest life. Disregard them and you'll be taking the long way home.' Are you then saying that those of us who encounter pain and suffering as we travel through life—and who doesn't encounter some hardships along the way?—have violated a natural law that has taken us off the freeway and onto one of those slower, more winding roads?"

"Look, Dar, as you have noted, every person on the planet will face good times and bad times—even if they live like saints. Painful events come to help us learn the lessons we need to learn at that point of our paths. Sad experiences arrive to help us heal, deepen and grow more philosophical. No one can avoid them because no one is perfect. So, being imperfect, even if we are living kind, noble and bold lives, means we still have many lessons to learn, right?"

"Makes perfect sense," I said with a grin, playing off Julian's words.

"So even the most awakened among us will still face pain and suffering because these experiences come to offer the specific lessons needed to rise to the next level of understanding and evolution. 'There are no mistakes, no coincidences. All events are blessings given to us to learn from,' said Elisabeth Kübler-Ross. Do you now see why pain and suffering are both wonderful and necessary?"

"Yes."

"One sage said it brilliantly when he recognized that life is like a river with two banks. On one bank we will find happiness and on the other we will see sorrow. As we move along the river, we will inevitably brush up against both banks. The real trick is not to stay stuck on either one too long."

"That's good. I like that metaphor a lot, Julian. So no one has a life without problems and sadness because these things come to teach us lessons and each of us, no matter how evolved we are, have lessons to learn?"

"Right. The only people without problems and adversity are six feet under the ground. To live is to face problems, pain and suffering. These things are vehicles for growth, expansion and lifelong learning. Life's trials are nothing more than opportunities to collect wisdom and platforms to remember more of our authentic power, if we choose. But let's not forget, every life will have its share of triumphs and beautiful times as well.

No hardships ever last. No setbacks are forever. No misery lasts an eternity. It may seem as though they will never go away as we experience them but that's not the truth. Life has its seasons, its chapters, if you will. And the hard times are ultimately the times that sculpt us into something better. The real point to take away though is that *if we choose to pay attention to these natural laws I speak of and live out our lives in a way that respects them deeply, we will spend a lot more time on the expressway than on those detours that are filled with challenges and pain. In this way, we clearly can minimize the amount we suffer.*"

"So, if suffering comes to teach us lessons that we need to learn, such as 'be a better person' or 'stop playing small with your life,' if we understand these truths or 'laws' as you call them, there is no need for us to learn them in painful ways. We'll experience less suffering in our lives, because suffering only happens when we are out of alignment with the laws that run the world. So we *can* have a dramatic influence on the way our lives unfold."

"Excellent, Dar!" exclaimed Julian as he raised his fist into the air with happiness. "But remember, you still might experience hardship because, being imperfect as we are, there will always be lessons for you to learn and sometimes these lessons need to come in ways that hurt. That's just the way it is. But yes, we can reduce the suffering in our lives by assuming absolute personal responsibility for ourselves and making wise choices during the hours of our days. In this way, we do shape our destiny and have the power to live much happier lives."

"Oh," Julian continued as he walked over to the CD player and began looking through the CD cases that sat atop it, "*the universe is not ignorant of your heart's longings.* The part of the plan that has been written for you would never involve you doing something that was wrong for you. The whole idea is for you to be happy. Your destiny will never lead you to do something that would make you unhappy to do. If you love doing business, the plan for you will probably not be for your life's work to be centered on being a doctor or becoming an actor. If a person loves being a writer—her heart soars when she's alone in front of her computer, writing with great conviction and passion as if nothing else mattered—her soul's purpose will not likely be for her to become a door-to-door salesperson. *The universe really does want you to win. The plan is for you to be very happy indeed.*"

Julian showed me some of the CDs he had collected, like a child might share his favorite toys with a good friend. There was Morcheeba's *Parts of the Process,* Coldplay's *A Rush of Blood to the Head,* a Bon Jovi bestseller and two I'd never seen before: one from a group called Our Lady Peace entitled *Gravity* and another by Lloyd Cole called *The Negatives.*

"Pretty eclectic musical tastes, Julian. You must be the hippest monk on the planet."

That made him laugh. His whole face lit up. "It's like I told you, Dar, music makes my soul sing. It's one of the sweetest pleasures of my life. I spend a lot of time in music stores and bookshops. Music and books. Two of my greatest pleasures."

On Julian's unmade bed were three books that looked tattered from many readings: *Meditations* by Marcus Aurelius, *The Greatest Salesman in the World* by Og Mandino and the curiously titled *The Saint, The Surfer and The CEO*—the titles some of these authors dreamed up never ceased to amaze me! He had few clothes in the room. His knapsack sat in the corner. There was no doubt that Julian lived simply.

Julian set aside a pair of khaki shorts, a white T-shirt and a pair of sandals. I saw that he had bought the sandals from The Gap. It was becoming increasingly clear to me that while Julian had few possessions and traveled through life lightly, he was not one of those spiritualists who shunned the real world and felt that the only route to enlightenment was to become an ascetic. He made no apologies for his love of the pleasures this world has to offer. His overall philosophy, to me, seemed very balanced. Balance head with heart. Balance chasing dreams and making things happen, with letting things happen and trusting in the higher plan. Balance an awareness that the purpose of life is to return to our spiritual selves with an appreciation that we are human beings with various imperfections, who reside in a world with many lovely pleasures that can—and should—be savored without guilt. *Ultimately, it seemed to me that Julian believed the golden key to a beautiful life was to balance Heaven and Earth. And that felt right to me.*

Julian reached for the Og Mandino book and pointed to a line that had been highlighted in yellow ink. "Here, read this jewel of truth, amigo." The line was simple, as I'd just learned all truths are. It read: "I am not on this earth by chance. I am here for a purpose and that purpose is to grow into a mountain, not to shrink to a grain of sand."

"Thank you, Julian," I said softly. "Thank you for saving my life."

# CHAPTER 4

# The Seeker Learns of the Crime of Self-Betrayal and How to Unchain Himself

*Cherish your visions; cherish your ideals; cherish the music that stirs in your heart, the beauty that forms in your mind, the loveliness that drapes your finest thoughts, for out of them will grow all delightful conditions, all heavenly environment; of these, if you remain true to them, your world will at last be built.*
　　　　　　　　　　　　—James Allen, *As You Think*

*How can you hesitate? Risk! Risk anything! Care no more for the opinion of others, for those voices. Do the hardest thing on earth for you. Act for yourself. Face the truth.*

　　　　　　　　　　　　—Katherine Mansfield

Julian knew I was deep in thought and he left me alone for a few moments, as if to allow me to process all that he had offered. While he went into the bathroom, I pondered the way that I had conducted my life all these years. I could hear him singing as the water from the tap flowed. A great sense of regret began to well up inside me as I reflected on the many mistakes of my past. Rather than using these mistakes to my advantage, as fodder for growth and learning, I had been asleep to the lessons they carried, walking through life blind to the opportunity for growth and wallowing in self-pity. I felt sad that I had not been exposed to Julian's philosophy at a much earlier age and lived a life that was more closely aligned with the natural laws he spoke of. So many precious years had slipped away, years I could have spent walking the path to my best and most true life rather than squandering the talents and gifts I'd been given on a life that was lived to please the expectations of others. I'd been swallowed up by the crowd, and had almost allowed it to destroy me.

When Julian returned, he put his arm around me. He could tell what I was going through. "'Forgiveness is the fruit of understanding,' said the wise monk Thich Nhat Hanh. You are exactly where you are meant to be on your path. As that understanding—and your awareness of the way life unfolds—grows, a beautiful sense of self-forgiveness will appear within you. You are far too hard on yourself," Julian said gently, surprising me by the depth of his intuitive power.

He led me out of the room, into the hallway. Beautiful art hung on the walls and lounge music flowed softly from a series of well-hidden speakers. It seemed as though most of the hotel's guests were still asleep.

"Tell me more, Julian," I said, gathering myself and feeling ready to hear more of the profound wisdom my brilliant, if unorthodox, life coach was sharing with me.

"Good enough, amigo," he replied as we walked into the

elevator. "A person who plays his biggest game as a human being—that is, lives according to his largest potential and walks the path of his authentic mission—is a person who is in love with himself," he said. *"Living an excellent life is a manifestation of self-love."*

"I've never considered that," I said.

"Someone who conducts his life as if he were one of the greatest people on the planet—a true heavyweight—is someone who not only has enormous self-respect but one who has deep respect for the force of nature that created him. There's a lot of talk these days about 'living in the moment' and 'savoring the now.' Don't get me wrong, that kind of thing is *essential* to living well. I believe in it and espouse it completely. You've even heard me talk that kind of talk in our short time together. *But it's all a balance,* and there's absolutely nothing wrong with also making time to reach for the stars and let the talents within you shine in a *big* way. *As a matter of fact, when you set big goals and chase big dreams, you are engaging in a hugely creative act. You are using your imagination and your abilities to build something wonderful. That's creativity in action."*

"Nice insight. I never really thought of going after my most meaningful goals as a creative act. But it is, isn't it? Doing so involves creating something from nothing more than the initial idea. Building a new business or launching a new product or chasing a real passion is no different than what an artist does as she transforms the vision in her mind into a beautiful work of art."

"Yes. And as we create the lives of our dreams, guess who we model?"

"No idea."

"We model the infinitely powerful force that created the entire world. Call that force 'God,' 'the universe' or 'Nature'—the label you put on it is just a word and I don't want to get hung up on labels. The point is that when you go after what you want, with love and wild abandon, you tap into the energy that created the stars and the seas. A kind of magic begins to enter your life and things happen that defy your comprehension. Signs start to appear, suggesting that you are on the right track. You are driving home and drive through ten green lights in a row, just as you are wondering whether the person you just courageously asked out on a date is the right one for you. Or the right person happens to call you at the right time, helping you decide if the job you were struggling with is the best one for you. Or the ideal solution to a difficult problem appears in a book you just happened to pick up while you were sitting in your dentist's waiting room, ready to have your teeth cleaned. What's that old expression: *'Synchronicity is God's way of remaining anonymous.'*"

"Oooh, that's a good one, Julian."

"Don't I know it," he said with smooth confidence as we walked out of the elevator and into the gleaming lobby. Sun poured through the floor-to-ceiling glass windows and the gerbera daisies that filled the lobby gave the space a magnificent feel. I was proud of this hotel and what it stood for. I felt good about what I'd created here.

"When you do your best and dedicate yourself to excellence, the universe supports you and puts wind beneath your wings. It sees a human being who is reaching for his ideals and trying to become what he was meant to be. That kind of effort never goes unnoticed by the eyes that watch over the world. Now, remember, not everything will work out the way you want it to. There's a higher intelligence at play whose logic we often cannot understand. But if you just keep doing your best and letting life do the rest, accepting whatever comes, with the knowledge that it's for your highest good, life will work out wonderfully. Better than expected, actually."

Just as I was letting that insight sink in, Julian got down on the floor of the lobby and started doing some strange maneuvers. The front desk team began to look and then giggle quietly. Maria was entranced. Julian ran his own race, that's for sure. He paid little attention to what others thought of him. It seemed so clear that so long as what he did felt true to him, he would do it. He lived life on his own terms. And as he had taught me, that was the *real* meaning of success.

"I'm doing the downward facing dog. Yoga is one of the practices I use each day to keep me energized and in good physical condition. You ought to try it. It's been around for thousands of years for a reason: it works. Hey, if Madonna and Sting swear by it, it can't be so bad, can it?" he said with a grin, as he focused in the posture, his muscles rippling as he moved gracefully.

After he had held the pose for a few moments, he rose to his feet and continued. "Anyway, back to my point. Too many spiritualists in our world today suffer from a disease I call 'spiritual apathy.' They will tell you not to chase your dreams or play too big, saying that this is controlling your destiny and forcing outcomes. What nonsense!" said Julian as he waved his arms in the air with dramatic flair.

"Yes, as I hope I've made clear all along, those who are living their best lives—the lives their destinies wished for them—have managed to strike a delicate balance between making it happen and *letting* it happen. I agree that trying *too* hard is nothing more than pushing the river and forcing outcomes. But too many spiritual seekers seem to believe that working hard, being disciplined and going for what you want is unhealthy and unspiritual. Nothing could be farther from the truth. Setting goals, managing your time well and taking calculated risks to get what you want is actually *very spiritual* because you are applying the talents and power that have been invested in you for a worthwhile cause. People who believe otherwise may be at the other extreme from the workaholics of this world, but their views are still extreme and unbalanced. And as far as I am concerned, extremism in any form is unhealthy."

"Is it possible for a person to be *too* spiritual?"

"Sure. Staying in your room and meditating or praying all day for the life of your dreams is not going to give you the life of your dreams and believing differently is nothing more than engaging in magical thinking. It's delusional actually. I told you that I believe there is a rough plan in place for our destinies—it was written before we were born into this world. Having said that, human beings have been given free will for a reason: *to take the steps required to bring our destinies to life.* There are lots of blanks we have the power to fill in and lots of dots to connect. You must put in the effort and make the sacrifices required to live the life of your dreams. You must be disciplined and make wise choices. Actions have consequences and to reap the harvest you dream of, you must sow the seeds. That's another of nature's laws. And if you don't believe me, just talk to any successful farmer. They will tell you that nothing grows in their fields without hard work and diligent seed-planting. If they just sat around meditating or praying all day, they'd lose the farm."

"That feels right to me," I said. "I can't imagine that my destiny will come knocking if I don't do anything to draw it to me. I agree with you, Julian, the more I think about it: we wouldn't have been given personal power, as human beings, if we were not meant to exercise it."

We walked outside, into the fresh air of the early morning.

"Exactly, Dar. Every gift we have been given—and every one of us has gifts—has been given to us for a reason. With each of the gifts we have received comes the responsibility that we sculpt it and develop it and then apply it out in the world in a way that enriches the lives of other people. People who are not willing to set an intention for all they want from life and then to *boldly* pursue it are ultimately people with much fear stirring within them. They are frightened. They have issues that need to be healed and shadows that need to be examined."

"What kinds of fears might be running them, Julian?"

"Fear of failure, fear of success, fear of the unknown, fear of rejection, fear of being different, fear of not being good enough . . . I could go on. Anyone who is not out there, doing their best, devoting themselves to playing their highest game and living at a standard of excellence is, at some root level, a person with fears within them in need of healing. Now, I need to be clear: there's not a soul on the planet who doesn't have some fear that limits him from living his truest potential.

Again, the very condition of being human is one of imperfection and much of this imperfection arises due to the fears we have picked up as we have left the perfection of our original nature and traveled out into the world."

"So all that talk by so many people these days about 'letting go of outcomes' and 'being present-centered' shows fear, right?"

"Not quite, Dar. The philosophy, in theory, is right *but the way they are executing it* is wrong. Remember the phrase I've been coaching you on: *do your best and then let life do the rest.* Chase your dreams. Do all you can to build the life you want. Visit the places that scare you and do not shrink from the greatness that you know in your heart you were meant to present to the world. And once you've done *everything* in your power, as a human being, to make your desires happen—*and only then*—let go of outcomes. After you've done your part of the equation by giving your all, relax and accept whatever comes back to you. You did all you could do. You acted responsibly and made the best moves and highest choices that were within your power to make. Now let the higher power take over and lead you to where you were meant to go. Let life take you to the path of your destiny. It is at this point that you need to just relax and surrender."

"Okay, I'm getting it. It's that balance thing again. I need to do my part and then life or nature or Infinite Intelligence or God, whatever label we want to put on the higher power that ultimately is in control, does the rest. And whatever comes, I should understand that it has come for a reason."

"It's actually come for your highest good and to take you

where you need to go. *If you've done your very best and lived in accordance with the laws of nature, whatever comes will be a blessing, even if it initially looks like a curse."*

"Very powerful ideas, Julian. Very powerful. So these so-called spiritualists and all their talk about letting go, living life without goals and surrendering to the moment are people who are, in truth, scared. They are playing small and letting their fears run their lives. They are out of balance," I observed, trying to distill and summarize what Julian had just taught me.

"Yes. For many of them, their 'spirituality' is nothing more than a mask they wear to protect the frightened little children within them who are running the show. They are afraid that they will fail or not be good enough or that the path might be difficult. So they make excuses to absolve themselves of any responsibility. They govern their lives by the position of the planets or by what some fortune-teller says is their fate. Don't get me wrong, Dar, I learned in India that astrology is a magnificent science that can be very reliable. It's been used with success for thousands of years. But it truly is all about a balance. To *completely* run my life by it is to play the game of the victim. To blame my moods, my inactions and my mistakes on the way the planets are aligned is to give away the power I have been given as a human being to the planets, the moons and the stars. It's a weak way to live. *Remember, you are not your moods but a force far bigger than them. You are not your psychology but a power far wiser than it."*

"What I hear you saying, Julian, is that, for someone not to do what's needed to go after the life they want, to the fullest extent of their human capacity, is actually *irresponsible* because they are not using the gifts they have been given."

"It's like I mentioned in the dressing room last night, 'Happiness is our birthright.' We have been hardwired to do extraordinary things with our lives and present exceptional gifts to the world. Martin Luther King Jr. said it well: 'Everyone has the power for greatness, not for fame but for greatness.' But we betray ourselves. We play small and timid with our lives. We buy into the belief system by which those around us teach us to govern our lives that says: 'do not dare,' 'do not dream,' 'do not shine too brightly or else you will stand out—and fail.'"

We walked out into the sunlight of a perfect day. The Ferrari was drawing admiring looks from many of the people arriving at the hotel. It was a stunning vehicle and appeared to be in immaculate condition, even though it was an older model. Julian smiled when he looked at it.

"Come on, amigo, let's go for a ride."

I'd never been in a Ferrari and was delighted by every aspect of the sensual experience it offered. As I relaxed into the tan-colored seats, I closed my eyes and luxuriated in the smell of rich Italian leather. When Julian turned the ignition, the engine roared to life. He shifted the car elegantly into first gear and sped away from the hotel as onlookers stared at the car and its two fortunate occupants.

Julian reached over and turned on the CD player. U2's *Beautiful Day* rang out from the superb sound system as we headed through the city's still-quiet streets and onto a freeway that would lead us into the countryside.

"Hey, Julian," I said. "Whose car is this anyway?"

"It's a secret," he replied simply as he tapped his fingers along with the music.

"Could you at least tell me where we're going?"

"The Camden Caves," Julian replied as he stepped on the accelerator. His eyes were completely focused on the road and his face reflected the joy that he was feeling. He clearly loved driving this car.

I'd heard of the Camden Caves. They were a series of ancient caves next to a waterfall that archeologists and adventurers alike frequently explored. I had no idea why Julian was taking me there. And I did not ask.

"It's time for me to start coaching you on The 7 Stages of Self-Awakening, Dar. Last night and earlier this morning was all a primer. You are doing beautifully—I know you will begin to see powerful results over the coming weeks and months. I can tell when I look into your eyes that you are committed. 'Commitment' is a very big and important word for me. Living a committed life is an incredibly important pursuit. 'Commitment' and 'accountability' are words that must flood the core of your being. You must think about these words often and devote yourself to standing by them."

"I promise I will take them seriously, Julian," I said with sincerity.

"The 7 Stages of Self-Awakening is a remarkably potent process for living your biggest life and walking the path to your destiny. The seven stages are a blueprint for awakening your best self and manifesting the potential that you have been given by the force that sent you into the world. Few people in the world today are aware of these seven stages, but that will soon change," said Julian with an air of mystery. "The seven stages reflect the pathway that every seeker needs to travel to return to his or her original nature—the state of mind, body and spirit that they first experienced when they were perfect and pure."

"And if I go through all seven stages, what will I be like as a person?" I wondered, hopefully.

"If you go through all seven stages, my friend, you will reach a state of being commonly referred to as 'enlightened.' Only a handful of people who have graced the planet before us have ever gone all the way to the end of this process, but that also is about to change. Once the world discovers this process for self-awakening that I am about to share, the world will change."

"That's an incredible promise, Julian."

"I know it is. I also know that while the system I'm about to share with you is simple to understand, the challenge comes in integrating it into your life. Now please don't get me wrong—I'm not saying that it's a difficult system to follow. Actually some parts of it are unbelievably easy. It's just that you will need to dedicate yourself to learning the process and staying with it until it becomes second nature."

"Okay, so what are The 7 Stages of Self-Awakening?" I asked.

"Stage One is the stage that most people on the planet are currently at. It's the stage of living an unconscious life—being asleep at the wheel, so to speak. This stage is known as 'Living a Lie' because people at this beginning platform of personal evolution are caught up in a lie about the way the world works and how they exist within it. Now I'm not, in any way, judging people who spend their entire lives at this stage. Who am I to judge another human being? But I am stating a fact when I tell you that this is the lowest level of consciousness that a person can operate at, when measured against all seven stages. You see, those of us who are at Stage One have no connection with the truth."

"What do you mean, Julian?"

"Well, over the coming weeks, I will share many truths with you as to how this world of ours operates and what you must do in order to find *authentic* success within it. To be unaware of the truths is to live a lie. To be unconscious as to what life is all about and why we are here is to be caught up in a misrepresentation. And sadly, that's the case for the vast majority of people on the planet. Like I told you last night, that's changing very quickly and there will be a quantum shift in the level of consciousness of most people soon. Did you see the movie *The Matrix*?" asked Julian.

"Yeah, I did. Pretty cool special effects," I acknowledged.

"Dar, that movie was about so much more than neat special effects. That's all that most people took from that movie. For many, it was just another Hollywood action film. But for the seekers among us—that is, for those of us searching for answers to the questions we have about why we are here and the true nature of the world—*The Matrix* was a philosophical masterpiece. It is a very deep movie. Actually, I'll go out on a limb and say that *The Matrix* is the most philosophical film ever made."

"Seriously?" I asked, surprised by Julian's statement.

"Absolutely. You see, as Morpheus explained to Neo in the film, this whole world of ours—the one we see through the eyes of our current level of perception—is nothing more than an illusion. It's a lie we tell—and sell—ourselves. Now, in the movie, everything the characters thought to be the real world turned out to be a computer-generated hallucination known as the Matrix.

That's the sci-fi, Hollywood part of the movie. This world of ours is not, of course, a computer-generated fantasy. But what you currently see as the real world, my friend, *is* just an illusion."

"I think you're losing me, Julian. What exactly do you mean when you suggest that the world I'm seeing is not what I think I'm seeing?"

"Well, the way you see the world is a function of the way you have been taught to see it. From the time you were a small child, you were trained and conditioned to believe certain things. For example, you were told to fit into the crowd and behave like everyone else. You were taught not to sing too loud when you were happy and not to dream too big when you were feeling inspired. You learned that those who are different would not be accepted and that conformity would lead to success. You were taught not to speak your truth and not to be too loving or else you'd be taken advantage of. You were taught that possessions and external power would bring you lasting happiness."

"Who taught us these beliefs?"

"Your parents. Your schoolteachers. Religious figures. Your friends. Television and the media."

"And what I was taught is untrue?"

"Well, there's a lot more going on in the world than most people are aware of. Or let me put it in a better way: You are not who you currently think you are. You have far more internal power and potential than you can imagine in your wildest dreams. You are destined for great things. And a lot of what you have been taught to believe about this big, beautiful world of ours is absolutely wrong."

"Like what?"

"First of all, *we are all connected at an invisible level. We are all brothers and sisters who belong to the same family. It's only an illusion that we are separate. Mystics and sages have told us that for thousands of years—we are all cut from the same cloth, and when you hurt another person, you hurt yourself as well.* This is one of the fundamental truths of nature and, yet, with the limited level perception available to people at stage one, most people can't see it. So we live a lie. We compete against each other for what we believe are scarce resources. We fail to support each other. We hoard and grab because we are in fear."

"In fear?"

"Yes, we fear that if another wins, we must lose. We fear that there just isn't enough abundance and prosperity in the world for everyone. We fear that if we genuinely help another person, we will somehow lose something rather than seeing the truth behind this lie which is that the more we help others, the more abundance will flood into our lives. One of the timeless truths of the universe can be stated simply: *When you shift from a compulsion to survive into a heartfelt commitment to serve, your life cannot help but explode into success.*"

"Powerful line," I observed.

"So stage one is all about this self-betrayal I've been hinting at since we first met. We were born into perfection—fearless, infinitely wise, of boundless potential and in a state of pure love. And, in our fear of not fitting in with the crowd, we begin to *forget* our original nature and adopt the beliefs, values and behaviors of the world around us. But look at the hatred in the world around us. The world has lost its way and is in the most sorry state it's ever been in. Too much fear and hatred on the planet today," Julian noted with some sadness. "It takes great strength to leave the crowd and be true to your original nature. But that's what leadership is all about—leaving the crowd and being true to who you really are. 'You don't find diamonds in storerooms, sandal trees in rows, lions in flocks and holy men in herds,' said the mystic Kabir."

"Why would anyone consciously betray themselves and begin to live a lie?"

"Excellent question. First let me say that when you do, in fact, betray yourself, the deeper part of you knows what you are doing. Each one of us has a witness—a deep place of knowing that lives at our authentic core—that watches *everything* we do. This place of knowing is commonly called a conscience. When we do not live authentically, the witness sees it. When we cheat or lie or act in selfish ways, the witness sees it. When we dishonor ourselves by playing small with our lives and refusing to live up to the magnificent potential that has been invested in us, the witness sees it. When we fail to pour love into the world, the witness sees it. All this betrayal of our true selves leads us to a slow and painful death. The witness cannot believe what we are doing to ourselves. It cannot believe that we are being so incongruent. It cannot bear to watch these kinds of crimes against our own humanity. So it begins to withdraw and shut down. We, as people, begin to lose self-respect. Our self-worth plummets. We begin to feel unhappy, angry and irritable. At a physical level we lack energy and vitality and may even grow ill. We do all this to ourselves but it generally happens at an unconscious level. We just buy into this lie about who we must be and how we must live. And it ends up killing us. Then, on our deathbeds, we finally understand that we did not live the lives we were meant to live. But, by then, it's too late."

"So why would anyone do this to themselves?" I pressed.

"Because we do not know better. It all starts when we are infants. And as infants, we look to our parents to teach us how the world works. We are hungry for their love. And so we do whatever we need to do to become like them, hoping that if we think, feel and act like them, we will receive their adoration. Unfortunately, in doing so, we leave our true selves behind."

"Self-betrayal," I stated.

"Exactly. So to awaken your best self, it's really a journey from where you now are—as an adult—to the place that you once knew—as a newborn. It's a journey home. It's a return to your original nature. We already are everything we've always dreamed of being. We've just forgotten it along the way. And that's why I believe the whole notion of self-improvement is nonsense. There's not one person on the planet who needs to improve—one cannot improve upon perfection and any suggestion that we need to do so only makes us feel more guilt about not being enough. *The duty of every human being is not self-improvement but self-remembering.* To self-remember is to reclaim the state of being and the authentic power that we lost when we left the ideal state of newborn children and walked out into this fear-filled world of ours, a world that spoiled us along the way."

"And this 'spoiling process,' if you will, has caused each of us to see an illusion. A filter gets set up between the truth of life and our human perception. This filter or personal context is comprised of all the lies we've been taught. The world we think we see, if we are living our lives at stage one of the process, is actually nothing more than a fantasy. It truly is a lie, of sorts.

What we are seeing is not the truth but a composite of all the ways we have been trained to see by those around us, well-meaning as they were."

"It's almost like we are a bunch of lab mice that have been conditioned to run on a treadmill for a little piece of cheese," I said.

"I'd agree with that. Remember, *we see the world not as it is but as we are*. We see the world though the filter of our personal perception, which comprises all the beliefs, fears, assumptions and values that we have assumed from our parents, early teachers and the world at large, in an effort to fit in with the crowd and be loved."

"Absolutely amazing, Julian. Hard to believe, actually. I've never, even once, stopped to think that the world I'm seeing as I go through my days just might not reflect the truth of what's actually happening."

"A while ago, I was coaching another individual and we were sitting in a classroom as I delivered the relevant lesson. He asked me a question and I gently gave him my answer. Instantly, his body language changed and he grew angry. Upon delving into what he believed caused this adverse reaction, he explained that he felt I had rejected him. The truth of the matter is that I did no such thing. As we went deeper into the source of his discomfort, he had a profound breakthrough. His father had been an exceedingly demanding person who often made my student feel like he was rejected. A belief had been set up within him that said 'people reject me' and this ancient pattern repeated itself throughout his life. Knowing this was extremely important for my student. Remember that awareness precedes choice and choice precedes change,"

Julian said as he turned off the freeway onto a single-lane road that led to the Camden Caves.

"What does that mean?"

"Once you become aware of something that's not right in your life, you can make new choices. And these new choices are what lead to positive changes. Let's say, for example, you have a scarcity mentality. You think you are the most generous person in the world but that's nothing more than denial. You don't want to look at what's really going on for you, beneath the surface. The truth of the matter is that you are very selfish and you try to keep everything you can for yourself. Everyone around you sees your selfish behavior. They can tell that you do not see the world as an abundant place, so you hoard. If they have done some work on themselves and have a certain level of personal evolution, they know that you are acting like this because, at some level, you are in fear. Fear of losing what you have, fear of being taken advantage of, fear of failure—the deeper issue is not important right now. But they can see that fear is driving your behavior and they know it comes from a childhood hurt—as all fears do, for every person on the planet. Anyway, you think of yourself as loving and generous. Now, let's say you have the courage to start asking people for honest feedback about how you could improve as a person. And let's say your loved ones are courageous enough to speak truthfully. They tell you what they have known all along: you operate from a perception of scarcity and you are not as giving as you have always thought yourself to be. If you listened to them, this would build new awareness in you. The shadows that were once within the realm of the subconscious would now move into the realm of the conscious where you could look at them. *Self-examination is the first step to personal greatness.* You could investigate where this belief system came from and where the fears first started. This new awareness, in turn, would lead to new choices, if you were willing to make them. You could be more giving and refuse to act in your old, selfish ways. These new choices would lead to new changes in the way you thought, felt and acted. And your life would then change. Nice little process, isn't it?"

"Very interesting, Julian. I know we are almost at the caves. Wow, this sure is a beautiful part of the world," I said, as I looked out at the lush meadows filled with yellow flowers. A stream ran alongside the road and an alley of oak trees lined the way. "What about the rest of the seven stages? Stage One is when people are unconscious to the truths of life and have little idea how the world really works. They are asleep to the fact that they project their own fears, false beliefs and biases out into the world and, as such, get a skewed vision of reality. I get that most people are at this stage and this is why the world is as messy as it is. We are divorced from our original nature. We have grown into false figments of our once magnificent selves. This self-betrayal has shut us down and given rise to self-loathing. My guess is that as we leave our loving, fearless and extraordinary selves and stuff ourselves into molds that allow us to fit into the crowd, we begin to hate ourselves at a deeper—perhaps subconscious—level. No wonder most people are so miserable and angry."

Julian began honking the horn. He raised one fist into the air while he kept the other on the steering wheel and started singing "It's a beautiful day" at the top of his lungs. He was once again pleased with my understanding of the wisdom and process he was sharing. I knew he was happy to be my coach and I was delighted to be his student. What I was learning from Julian was truly priceless. If more people could hear what I had been hearing, this world of ours really would be a very different place. It would be a place of greater justice, authenticity and love. In that moment, I committed to not only mastering the information I had been blessed to receive, I dedicated myself to spreading it to others. The term "evangelist" has taken on negative connotations these days. In truth, it simply refers to "one who spreads good news." I would spread Julian's message. I would become an evangelist.

Julian parked the car on a grassy slope and we began to walk along the path that would take us to the caves. He took off his sandals and walked barefoot. Julian did not say anything, instead preferring to hum a song while taking in the gorgeous gifts of nature that surrounded us. As we drew near to one of the caves, he began to speak.

"The first of the seven stages is 'Living a Lie.' Asking the right question evokes the right answer, you know? Questions offer powerful vehicles to promote self-awareness. Actually, that brings up a good little point: a great question to journal on when I'm not around is 'what things will I no longer tolerate in my life?' Anyway, I know you will no longer betray yourself and live a life that is not yours. Stage Two of the seven stages is known as 'The Choicepoint.' Once you grow aware that you are following the crowd and living an unauthentic life, you are presented with a choice."

"That's the part in *The Matrix* where Neo is given the choice between swallowing the blue pill or the red pill, right?

I'm beginning to see how deep and meaningful that movie really is, Julian. I need to see it again," I promised.

"Good idea. And you are right. Once you see that you have bought into the illusion the crowd wants you to believe is reality, you will have a choice: continue to live as you have always been living—and in so doing, resign yourself to a life of unhappiness and mediocrity—or take the red pill, so to speak, and step up to your biggest life. And never forget what poet David Whyte once observed: 'The soul would rather fail at its own life than succeed at someone else's.' Nothing's more important than having the bravery to live *your* life. Stage Three is called 'Awareness of Wonder and Possibility.' At this stage, you begin to see with a new set of eyes. You see more of the truth than you have ever seen before. You begin to understand that the world wants you to win and that it is a place of great abundance, opportunity and majesty. You also begin to see that people, at their core, are good and it is only because of the hurts that life has visited on them that they do bad things. I'm not saying that we all don't have choices—of course we do and everyone can choose to be kind, whole and good, no matter how much they have suffered. All I'm suggesting is that, at this stage, you begin to separate who people truly are from *their behavior*, which might present as hurtful and mean. You begin to see that people who act like this are in pain. No one with a wide open and happy heart could *ever* hurt another person. At this point along the process of self-awakening, you also become intimately aware of your best self. You see all the self-betrayal more clearly than ever and come to know what you are truly made of. This is an incredibly inspiring stage of the journey home."

"What's Stage Four?"

"Well, after you've left the stage of Living a Lie and passed
The Choicepoint by making the decision to awaken your best
self, and after you've become aware of the world beyond the
illusion—a world of extraordinary wonder and limitless possibility—you reach the fourth stage: 'Instruction from Masters.'
It is at this stage that the seeker usually begins to search for
various teachers and explores many different paths to learning. She is hungry for answers and healing. It can be a very
confusing time because when lots of new knowledge comes at
the seeker in a short space of time, it is hard to assimilate it all.
But please know that *confusion always gives rise to clarity*
over time and a moment does come when all the new learning
becomes wonderfully integrated within your understanding.
This is the beginning of *real* wisdom. After this comes Stage
Five: 'Transformation and Rebirth,' which can be the most
challenging stage. But it is also one of the most unforgettable.
It is at this stage that your biggest self starts to present itself
on a daily basis and your entire world begins to change. True,
change is not always easy, but the benefits that you will receive
at this point of the process will serve you well for the remainder of your life. Stage Six is 'The Trial.' Before a seeker
reaches her treasure, she will face a trial. The purpose of the
trial is twofold: first to ensure that she has learned all the
lessons she was meant to learn along the way and second, to
see how badly she wants the prize. It is at this stage that most
people give up. Too many people retreat at this point when,
sadly, had they persisted a little bit more, their greatest gift
would have been available just around the corner. And finally,
Stage Seven is 'The Great Awakening of Self.' To get to this

point—and few do, as I've suggested—you reach the state of enlightenment. You become all those things that reflect your original nature. You return to the way of being that you knew when you were connected to the force of nature that sent you into the world. You become fearless, innocent, infinitely wise, of boundless potential and pure love. No shadows—all light. You can get to that stage—if you are willing and *devoted*. But to get to this final place, you have to want to get there more than you want life itself. Makes me think of what Sheila Graham once wrote: 'You can have anything you want if you want it desperately enough. You must want it with an exuberance that erupts through the skin and joins the energy that created the world.'"

"Beautiful words," I applauded.

"And what better place could any human being ever aspire to reach than enlightenment?" asked Julian as we walked into a darkened cave. "Now I must tell you, The 7 Stages of Self-Awakening is not a magic-bullet, quick-fix kind of a process for personal transformation. It takes effort, patience and time to happen. Over the coming weeks, I'll take you through various experiences to bring the seven stages to life for you. I am your coach and it is my duty to show you the seven-stage process. But it will fall to you to live it over the weeks, months and even years that will follow my visit with you."

I felt a tinge of sadness within me. Julian had just entered my life last night and to speak so soon of his leaving was dismaying. In our short time together, he had already filled my heart with great inspiration and taught me so much wisdom. I knew that if I chose to act on even a small amount of the knowledge he had already given me, my whole life would assume a very different look.

Once again, Julian sensed my feelings.

"Hey, amigo, not to worry, we have big things to do together and I'm around for a while. And by the time I'm done with you, you won't need me. You'll be having too much fun on your own," he said with a healthy laugh.

Julian then took my arm and gently led me into the dark cave. After walking for about a minute, he asked me to sit down on the ground and stare at the wall in front of me. "Stay completely focused on that wall, Dar. Do not take your eyes off it. Promise?"

"I promise," I replied.

All of a sudden, the cave lit up. I had no idea what was going on behind me but I could hear Julian shuffling around. As I stared at the wall, I saw various images being projected on the rock face in front of me.

After about ten minutes of watching the objects dance across the wall of the cave, I heard Julian speak.

"What you are watching on the cave's wall is a mere illusion. It is a lie. Now it's time to see the truth. Are you willing?"

"Yes, I am," I said, still keeping my eyes on what was going on in front of me.

"Then turn around and see what's *really* happening."

I turned around and saw that Julian had lit a small fire. He also had, in his hands, a number of small stone objects that he was placing in front of the fire. These objects projected the images I was viewing on the cave wall in front of me.

"Ever read Plato's *Republic*, Dar?" asked Julian.

"No, never got around to it."

"It's important to read the great books first, you know. Otherwise, you just might find that you run out of time. Anyway, there is a section in the book in which a crowd of people are sitting in a cave, much like this one. This crowd is watching the images projected on the wall, much as you did. The sad thing is that, for their entire lives, they believed that what they saw was the truth; they never realized that they were only viewing an illusion. One day, one of the people from among the crowd dared to be different. He dared to become a seeker and he searched for the truth. He unchained himself from the ground and left the crowd by having the courage to see what was behind him, rather than continue to stare at the projected images in front of him. And what he saw shocked him."

"He saw a fire, I'll bet. And he saw that the images on the wall were mere projections of the objects being placed in front of the fire. He stopped believing the lie he had always believed and, for the first time in his life, he saw the truth."

"Perfect," Julian said, as he nodded his head with great satisfaction. "Perfectly noted. And that new awareness changed his life. Now that you've got my point, let's get out of here. It's a little creepy in this place if you ask me," he said with a chuckle. Julian put out the fire and we stumbled out of the cave, towards the light.

Julian led me down a path in a wooded area. The smell of pine and cedar brought back childhood memories of hiking in the woods with my father. Soon, I heard the sound of water. As we drew nearer, I saw a small waterfall, and above it, a rainbow.

"That's a good sign," said Julian happily. "Now, stand under the waterfall," he instructed.

"You're kidding!"

"No. I only need you to do it for a few minutes. It will cleanse you and serve as a metaphor for letting go of impurities you have collected since leaving your once-perfect state of being. Get under the waterfall and close your eyes. Imagine the water washing away all your limiting beliefs, false assumptions, fears and biases."

I did what Julian told me to do and, though the water was cold at first, the experience was amazing. I felt lighter, happier and more pure.

"You are now aware of the illusion under which you have lived your life," said Julian as I stepped into the sun to dry off. "You are now ready to stop lying to yourself and leave the crowd in search of the truth. Let go of the chains binding you to the ground and stand up for your biggest life. In doing so—in letting go of the lie and living the life meant for you—you will find something every one of us craves: *freedom*. You are now ready to leave Stage One of The 7 Stages of Self-Awakening."

Julian then asked me to close my eyes and sit on a grassy bank next to the waterfall. "These are the words of the great author Herman Hesse, and I want you to commit them to heart, Dar. They speak to what you've learned this morning." Julian spoke in a loud voice, as if to proclaim to all of nature the truth of what he was uttering:

*"It is time to come to your senses. You are to live and to learn to laugh. You are to learn to listen to the cursed radio music of life and to reverence the spirit behind it and to laugh at its distortions. So there you are. Nothing more will be asked of you."*

# CHAPTER 5

# The Seeker Discovers the Single Most Important Choice a Human Being Can Make

*I know of no more encouraging fact than the ability of a man to elevate his life by conscious endeavor. It is something to paint a particular picture, or to carve a statue, and so make a few objects beautiful. It is far more glorious to carve and paint the very atmosphere and medium through which we look. This morally we can do.*

—Henry David Thoreau

We were leaving the wilderness where I had completed the first stage of The 7 Stages of Self-Awakening. Julian was once again at the wheel of the red Ferrari.

"Every true seeker on the path to awakening and self-realization eventually reaches a place where he will be presented with the opportunity to make a choice that will dramatically alter his life forever. Sometimes this turning point is brought on through intense suffering such as the loss of a loved one, an illness, a financial crisis or a tragic accident. At other times, it will surface simply because the seeker is ready to get to the next level of living and has done the advance inner work required to make this a possibility," offered Julian as he took a sharp turn onto one of the highways that would lead us back into the downtown core. "If you have left Stage One of The 7 Stages of Self-Awakening by becoming aware of the self-betrayal you have been engaging in, you cannot help—as a seeker of the truth and an explorer of your biggest life—but reach Stage Two: The Choicepoint."

"And my guess, Julian, is that the way the seeker shows up at this Choicepoint, in many ways, determines his destiny. Make one decision and you get to ride one of those freeways you taught me about earlier. Take another and you ride the bumpier routes."

"Yes, that's right, Dar. The true decision you will face at The Choicepoint comes down to either showing a heartfelt willingness to advance confidently on the conscious path to your authentic life, or a regression to the life you once lived, a return to the waking sleep you once knew. *Ultimately, The Choicepoint offers you the chance to choose your biggest life or to stay small and remain among the herd of lemmings, unconsciously following those around you as each in turn falls off the cliff. I'll tell you one thing from personal experience: if you do not make the higher and more noble of the two decisions that present themselves at The Choicepoint, you will be setting yourself up for a life of deep regret and utter heartbreak by the time you reach the end.* Nothing so destroys the heart as the knowledge that you had the chance to manifest the gorgeous potential that you were meant to be and you refused to accept the call. *To refuse to accept the call of your best life is to insult the force that created you,*" Julian stated, with even greater intensity than usual. Suddenly, he pulled off the freeway onto a side road that led to a small community hospital located in a suburb of the city.

"Why are we going in here, Julian?" I asked, somewhat confused. Julian's coaching never ceased to be rich with adventure and suspense.

"You'll see," came the prophetic reply.

As we walked in through the main reception area of the hospital, two attractive nurses rushed over to greet Julian. "Hey, honey," one of them said flirtatiously, "nice of you to stop by to say hello." The other grinned as she teased, "Hi, Julian. Finally decided to have that physical?" Both of them erupted into laughter and gave my one-of-a-kind life coach a warm hug. "Seriously, Julian," the one who had spoken first said, "It's great to see you again. Go on up, they're expecting you."

"Could you keep an eye on my friend for a second, ladies?" asked Julian. "I need to pop into the gift shop for a minute."

While Julian went off to do his errand, I tried to figure out what was going on. I needed some answers.

"How do you both know Julian?" I asked.

"Oh, he comes here nearly every day," one of them said. "He's our best volunteer," the other chimed in. "Everybody loves Julian. He walked into this place one day, just a few weeks ago, as a matter of fact, and said he wanted to help out. Specifically asked to be placed in the terminal care ward. I still recall him saying something about 'needing to be an instrument of service and adding value to human beings.' Julian's quite an idealist, you know?"

"I know," I responded with a nod.

Julian returned with a huge bouquet of flowers in his arms. "Come on, Dar, there's a special group of people I'd like to introduce you to."

We walked down a long corridor with sterile white walls. The whole place smelled of ammonia and coffee. At the end of the hallway was a lounge. As we entered it, the six people sitting within it immediately stood up to greet Julian with smiles and hugs. It was clear they held Julian in enormously high regard. It was also clear that Julian was moved by their generous display of affection. I detected tears in his eyes. He saw what I saw.

"There's nothing wrong with a man crying," he whispered into my ear. "Never forget that. A person closed off from his feelings lacks sensitivity, compassion and empathy. Such people are of the kind who start wars, commit crimes and spread hate. Do not avoid your feelings, Dar. They are an essential part of the authentic person that you are."

Now Julian spoke aloud to the group gathered in front of us. "These ladies and gentlemen are my friends," he said. "Ladies and gentlemen, please say hello to my friend Dar." Each of them warmly shook my hand. I was asked to sit down, which I did.

"We've been expecting you, Julian. Is this the man you asked me to speak to?" asked a man who appeared to be in his eighties. He wore a checkered suit with a white shirt and a bowtie. His thinning gray hair had been neatly slicked back.

"Yes, Peter, this is the man. Why don't you share with him what you shared with me a week or so ago when I came in to visit you. Your words were very powerful. I wanted him to hear them from you."

"Well," said the elderly man, "I just told our young friend Julian here that now that I am at the end of my life, my greatest regret is not letting the music within me sing. I know, deep in my heart, that there was a song inside of me that needed to be expressed," he said poetically. "There was a creative mission hidden in me that called out to be liberated and realized. What I mean is that we all have special things we are meant to do with our lives. Each and every one of us is a special creature, endowed with miraculous capacities and unbelievable abilities."

"Peter here used to be a motivational speaker before he ended up in this place," one of the women kidded. The whole group began to laugh. It's been said that laughter is the shortest distance between human hearts. When we laugh together, all the social constructs that keep us apart fall to the wayside and we connect as real people. It's a beautiful thing to behold. It was in that moment that I realized the truth of one thing Julian had told me: we are all brothers and sisters of the same family. We are all bonded together at an invisible level and a voice of knowing within me told me that to disregard this truth was to buy into the illusion fostered by the crowd. We are not separate, I appreciated. We *are* connected with unseen ties. Even more so than through laughter, I have since discovered that we can connect with each other through the common sharing of our pain. If everyone in the world came together for half an hour and shared all of the personal suffering they have endured over the course of their lives, we would all be friends. There would be no enemies. There would be no wars.

The old man continued. "As I was saying, *my greatest regret is not listening to myself.* I knew I could do great things in my life. I was a very good writer when I was younger; I had even won some literary prizes during my university days. But my mother wanted me to be an accountant. She said that if I didn't listen to her, it would be the mistake of a lifetime. Actually, the mistake of my lifetime was not being true to myself and doing what I felt I was meant to do. So now—and you should know that the doctors in here tell me that I probably only have a few weeks left—I am so sad at the choice I made. I feel I've wasted my whole life. Eighty-seven years have gone by in a flash. It feels like it was just yesterday that I got married to my bride, Margaret. It feels like just yesterday that I watched my children being born. Now Margaret's dead and my children have gone off to lead lives of their own. Your life will whiz by quicker than you could ever imagine. The days will slip into weeks, the weeks into months and the months into years. You look pretty young now, but watch out—you'll look like me before you know it. Life's like that. So live the life that you are meant to live. Your life is far too important to wait until you are just about to die to wake up. I lived my mother's life when I should have had the wisdom to live my own. I spent my life trying to please others. But where are they now? All those people I lived to please are no longer around. *On your deathbed, the only person you'll have to answer to is the person you look at in the mirror every morning. You'd better be true to him.* I committed 'the crime of self-betrayal,' to use Julian's phrase. That's what's really going to kill me. Not the cancer."

The room fell completely silent. Peter's friends looked down, each apparently feeling sadness on not only hearing the tale of another man's deepest regret in life, but on being reminded that he would soon no longer be with them. *Life is such a fragile thing. I never truly knew that until now. It is a priceless treasure that we are given to guard and make use of to the best of our ability. That it will not come again is what makes it so sacred.* And yet, most people who live among the crowd never press the pause button in their lives and stop for even sixty seconds to reflect on why they are here and what they are meant to do.

After we left the Camden Caves, Julian had shared a little story with me. A wise sage met a beggar on the street one day. The beggar, not knowing to whom he was speaking, stopped the sage and asked him three questions: Why are you here? Where are you going? Is there an important reason that you are going there? The sage looked at the beggar and asked how much money he generally made on a given day. On hearing the honest answer given to him, the sage said, "Please come and work for me. I will pay you ten times that amount if only you will ask me these three questions before I do my meditation, early each and every morning."

I've since learned that reflection is the mother of wisdom. We must carve out some time each day to ask ourselves why we are here, how we are living and whether we are making the highest use of the gifts that life has given us. We must pay attention to life. We must frequently be in connection with our dreams. This universe of ours really is a friendly place and we would not be able to dream a dream without having the corresponding capacity to bring the dream to life. "The universe wants us to win," Julian often said. "We just need to get out of our own way."

Peter's comments touched me deeply. I knew that's what Julian hoped would happen. I needed to make some decisions. I needed to take a stand for my biggest life, once and for all.

We spent about half an hour at the hospital, drinking herbal tea and sharing stories with the lovely people Julian had befriended. Julian also spent a few moments arranging the fresh flowers in the room for them. He was a man of extraordinary compassion and sensitivity. We thanked them for their hospitality and then the group walked with Julian and me out to the Ferrari. Everyone really did love Julian. And everyone adored that car.

"So as you continue along this path to your authentic life—as you leave the crowd and begin to live by *your* values, *your* beliefs and *your* heart's desires, you, as a seeker, will *inevitably* reach The Choicepoint. How you respond at this juncture will make all the difference in terms of how the rest of your life will unfold," summarized Julian as we rolled out of the hospital's parking lot with my new friends waving goodbye to us. "Never forget what Harriet Beecher Stowe once wrote: 'The bitterest tears shed over graves are for words left unsaid and deeds left undone.' Become a person of action, one of those indomitable souls who goes out and hunts down his greatest life. Do the best that you know how to do. And then let go and accept whatever comes to you with a happy heart and perfect certainty that this is what nature intended for you."

"Got it, coach. Hey, you still haven't told me who owns this car. It's not yours, is it?"

"No, it's not mine. I travel too light these days to own something like this. I'm a very simple man. But it was mine," Julian admitted. "This was my old Ferrari."

"Really?" I exclaimed. "When I was a kid, my dad used to take me for drives through your neighborhood. I used to stare at this car all the time. Man, I loved this baby."

"I know," replied Julian. "I'd catch you looking at it from time to time," he said with a wink.

"Really?"

"Sure. An industrialist client of mine bought the car from me just before I left for India. He said I could buy it back from him if I ever wanted to—no questions asked. He also said I could drive it whenever I returned to the city. He's been very generous to me, in many ways. He's loaned it to me while I'm here."

We drove in silence for a long time. As we entered the hotel's driveway, Julian brought the car to a halt. The bellman smiled at both of us and gave me the thumbs-up sign. He appeared duly impressed.

"Open up the glove compartment, Dar—there's something in there for you. I want you to look at the present after I leave you, which, unfortunately, must be in a few minutes. I have a massage scheduled and I never like to be late for massage appointments. It's a regular gift I give myself."

"I'd never have guessed you'd be such a big fan of massages," I replied.

"Why not, Dar? Massage therapy is a wonderful way to

promote vitality, eliminate toxins and elevate overall health. I have a whole series of what I call 'success structures'—practices that I build into my week—that I rely on to keep me healthy, happy and in deep peace. Daily exercise, an elite performance diet, meditation, time spent in nature and a massage every seven days are things I do for myself so that I'll live a long time and be able to do the work I've been called to do. I have a mission in this life of mine and I intend to do it. A massage a week might seem expensive to some people but to me, it's an investment, not an expense. It's money well spent. I'm of no value to anyone if I'm lying in a hospital room. I just see my massages as a cost of doing business, so to speak."

"Interesting way to view it, Julian."

"Today's been a big day for you, Dar. I've planted some seeds that will flourish into some wonderful insights over time. Trust me on that one—you got some big pieces of learning today."

"I'm very grateful for this day with you, Julian. You shared some pretty profound lessons with me. I know that. And the way you shared them made them unforgettable. I had no idea learning could be so fun, memorable and moving."

"Learning should be fun, memorable and moving. Learning from books, intellectually, is great. But learning in a way that engages you at an *emotional* level is even more powerful and sustaining. That's why I try to set up experiences to help you learn what you need. Experience is always the best teacher. Anyway, nicely done today."

I opened up the glove compartment and found a gift-wrapped package inside. It was evident from the uneven edges that Julian had done the wrapping himself, but I gave him full marks for effort and thoughtfulness.

"Thanks, Julian. I can't imagine what's inside but I know I'll value it, coming from you."

"Oh, by the way, these are for you as well," he stated as he handed me the keys to the Ferrari.

"Do you want me to park the car?" I asked, willing to help Julian in any way I could.

"No, my friend," he paused. "The car's yours."

I was *stunned*. Was Julian really offering his former car to me? As I kid, I could not have imagined a better dream coming true. Even now, owning a classic Ferrari in immaculate condition was a notion that thrilled me.

"I don't want to manufacture The Choicepoint for you, Dar—one will intersect the path you are on—the journey of the seeker—naturally. As you continue to open your eyes in search of the truth, a Choicepoint will necessarily present itself. But I really want to do my best to bring The 7 Stages of Self-Awakening to life for you and so I've tried to create some memorable experiences that will teach you the essence of each stage. I'm now giving you a choice—and I'm totally serious: you can have this Ferrari, if you want it. My former client is perfectly fine with it. He said that whatever I want is whatever he wants. I've done him some very big favors in the past. But there is one little catch."

"Let's hear it," I said with a smile, fearing the worst.

"Well, if you make the choice to take the car, I can no longer be your coach. It's either this car or my coaching. We can still be friends, but I'll have to move on to my next assignment. You see, that's what The Choicepoint is all about: making some kind of a sacrifice. Nothing good comes without some kind of sacrifice. The Choicepoint is all about leaving the world you have known and venturing out onto the unknown frontiers of your highest life. And to access that highest life, you have to want it more than anything else in the world. You have to want it more than even this Ferrari. Most people believe that it takes months and years to transform their lives. Actually, you can literally change your life in an instant, by making a single decision never to go back to the way you have been living— no matter what. What takes the months, years and sometimes decades is the *maintenance* required to abide by that decision."

"Nice distinction, Julian," I said.

"So it's your choice, amigo: this rare and exotic sports car or the chance to be true to yourself. It's completely up to you."

"Oh, Julian," I replied with a sigh. "You're killing me, man," I added with a laugh. "You know what my answer is—I'm no fool. I'll take the coaching. I'll choose my biggest life!" I exclaimed.

Julian clapped his hands, delighted with my decision. "As far as I'm concerned, that's the only choice to make at The Choicepoint—the choice to reach for the stars and advance towards the life that has been destined for you. But, I'll tell you what, since you've been such a good sport about things, I'll make you another offer. If you don't mind dropping this car off at my friend's home, you can take it for a spin around the city. Deal?"

"Deal."

Julian gave me a hug and exited the car. Then he popped his head back in. "Let's meet back here seven days from now, at five A.M. sharp, please. I want to explain Stage Three of The 7 Stages of Self-Awakening to you. You'll love what you learn. Until then, be gentle with yourself. You are going through a lot of change, so make time for lots of self-care activities. Go for long walks in the woods. Listen to your favorite music. Get a massage. And of course, find the time to experience silence, stillness and solitude. You're doing great. I'll see you soon, my friend."

And with those instructions, the former superstar lawyer turned all-knowing monk and sage life coach walked into The Q Hotel and out of sight. I remained in the passenger seat of the Ferrari for a long time, reflecting on the day and committing from the deepest place within me to keep walking the conscious path of life. I unwrapped Julian's gift. It was a brand new copy of Plato's *Republic*. As I flipped through the pages, I saw Julian's writing on two of the blank pages at the front. Here's what it said:

*Dear Dar,*

*First, let me honor you for your bravery. It takes great resolve and power to leave the gravitational forces of the crowd and begin to live more truly. The space shuttle uses more fuel during its first three minutes after takeoff than it requires during the remainder of its orbit around the entire earth for this same reason: there is a pull exerted by the world that takes great energy to overcome. But overcome it you must, my friend, to avoid a life of regret and sadness.*

*By the time you look through this book, you will have already made the single greatest choice of your life: to walk the path of your destiny and reach for your greatest life (I knew you would make that choice—your father was a wise and great man and the fruit never falls very far from the tree). I'm now inviting you to make some daily choices that will help you play your biggest game as a human being. These are five essential practices to integrate into your life over the coming weeks and months if you really want to live the beautiful life that's meant for you. I call these The 5 Daily Devotions:*

1. *Devote yourself to rising at 5 A.M. each and every morning. Those who get up early are those who get the best from life.*
2. *Devote yourself to setting aside the first sixty minutes of your day as your "Holy Hour." This is your sacred time to do the inner work required to help you become your best. Use this period to read from the wisdom literature, to meditate or pray, to reflect on the state of your life and the progress of your dreams in your journal or to think deeply about what must unfold over the coming hours of the day in order for you to feel it was a successful one. Performing this ritual daily will help you to shine brightly in the world and live at your highest.*
3. *Devote yourself to displaying a standard of care, compassion and character well beyond what anyone could ever imagine from you. In doing so, you will be doing your part to aid in the building of a new world.*
4. *Devote yourself to displaying a standard of excellence at work far higher than anyone would ever expect from you. Abundance and fulfillment will flow back to you.*

5. *Devote yourself to being the most loving person you know and thinking, feeling and acting as though you are one of the greatest people currently on the planet (because you are). Your life will never be the same and you will bless many lives.*

*Let me close by telling you that I admire you, as a man. You have been through a lot and far brighter times are coming—as they always do. "In every Winter's heart lies a quivering Spring. Behind the veil of each night waits a smiling dawn," wrote the wise poet Kahlil Gibran. You know he was right.*

*Your fan . . . Julian*

I had no doubt that the happiest seasons of my life were still in front of me. I had no doubt that my best was yet to come.

# CHAPTER 6

# The Seeker Walks into Wonder and Possibility

*With life I am on the attack, restlessly ferreting out each pleasure, foraging for answers, wringing from it even the pain. I ransack life, hunt it down.*

—Marita Golden

*The World is a great book, of which they who never stir from home read only a page.*

—St. Augustine

In the week since my last visit with Julian, profound shifts had begun to occur. I began to feel differently, sensing that I was beginning to live life on my own terms and with far greater consciousness than ever before. I was paying attention to the choices I was making in terms of how I thought, felt and acted and ensured each of these came from a place of impeccable integrity and genuine honor. This, in turn, led to me feeling more confidence and inner peace than I had experienced in my entire life. In many ways, I felt unstoppable. I felt alive. I felt so much joy. I felt I was becoming a better version of myself. I knew I was awakening.

However, to be truthful, many fears began to surface. A seeker on the path home to his or her authentic and biggest self will always have to face fears they never knew existed. While living an unconscious life, many of our fears live within the realm of our subconscious minds. Consciously, we do not even know they are there. But they are, affecting every one of our choices and running our lives at an invisible level. As we awaken and choose to see our lives from a more truthful frame of reference, our fears begin to see the light of day—and we must confront them. This is usually a scary thing.

But I've learned that our fears are straw monsters. If we deny them, they remain in the basement, secretly sabotaging our lives and keep us running away from our dreams. But if we confront them, by inviting these scary monsters upstairs for a cup of tea—if we get to know them—we realize they were so much smaller than we first thought. Just as a shadow fades when brought into the sunlight, a fear invited into the light of our human awareness begins to evaporate. You see, what we resist will persist. And if we refuse to do the inner work required to look at and then work through our fears, they will always run us. But if we have the courage to self-explore and get to know our fears, they will move through us, and then be released. What we resist will indeed persist. What we befriend, we inevitably will transcend.

Julian once told me of a story about a mountain climber who reached the summit of the peak he was scaling at midday. The challenge then became getting back down, to a place of safety, before the sun had set. As he descended, he noticed the sun getting lower and lower. He quickened his pace but, as the hours slipped away, the light faded and the sun sank lower on the horizon. He began to grow frightened and many fears began to surface. He felt that if he did not get to the bottom of the mountain, he would be caught midway and be placed in an extremely dangerous position, perhaps even falling to his death.

Finally, the sun set and the climber found himself in utter darkness. Desperate, he fumbled to find something he could hold on to, eventually clinging to a branch that grew from a crevice in the stone face of the mountain. The climber spent the night hanging on to that branch, frozen with fear, believing that if he let go of it, he would fall to his death on the rocks below. The night was a nightmare for him—pure terror.

But when the first rays of the morning cast light once again, he began to laugh. He could not believe what he saw. *His fear was only an illusion.* Only six inches below him rested a ledge. In the darkness, he could not see it. But in the light, he realized that all he had to do was go six inches lower and he could have spent the entire night in safety and relative comfort. His fears were unfounded. His terror had no basis in reality. And fears, I have learned, are like that. They keep us small, shackled; they spoil our lives. And yet every single one of the fears that limits us is truly only six inches deep. Do not let these fears own you. Do not let them spoil your life.

I arrived at The Q precisely at 5 A.M. It had become much easier to get up early and I was enjoying the extra hours the discipline of early rising offered me. As suggested by Julian, I would use this "base camp" time at the front end of my day to plan, visualize, contemplate and read from the great books of wisdom. This connected me to the essential truths that lay at the foundation of every great life. Reading each morning also inspired me, reminding me that no life, no matter how wonderful, is free of problems and challenges. The only individuals without any problems are those in their graves. Actually, it is the existence of problems and challenges that makes us bigger, stronger and wiser. We can run from them, and become bitter, complaining that life is hard. Or we can embrace them, and become better. It is generally in the times of our greatest pain that we are most intimately connected with who we truly are—and were meant to be. Martin Luther King Jr. once said: "The ultimate measure of a man is not where he stands in moments of confidence but where he stands at times of challenge and controversy."

As I walked through the lobby doors, I saw Julian chatting with the front desk staff. He had them laughing and he was chuckling along with them. Just hearing him laugh made me laugh. His laughter was so pure, real and childlike. I had never met anyone like Julian. He was so genuine and had no façade. He seemed, to me, to be the kind of person that each one of us wants to become: playful, loving, wise—and fearless.

I was surprised to see that Julian had his robe on today. I had expected him to dress informally again, but was delighted by his attire and the splendor that it reflected. I sensed that Julian was proud to wear this traditional dress of the Sages of Sivana. I also got the feeling that wearing the robes not only reminded him of his chosen path, it reminded him of them.

"Good morning, amigo," he bellowed from across the lobby. "Just having some fun with these early risers over here.

Important club we all belong to, you know. Nothing like having some discipline in your life to make it a big and beautiful one."

"I hear you, Julian. I'm getting used to it."

"Well, great," he said as he walked over and put one of his bronzed arms around me with great affection. "I missed you, you know."

"I missed you too, Julian. That was quite a day we had last week. I can't wait to see what today's coaching session is all about."

"Today you will learn about Stage Three of The 7 Stages of Self-Awakening, Dar. Stage Three is all about seeing with a new set of eyes. You see, my friend, most people on the planet today are walking through life blindly, just following the crowd. They are living a lie. They think they see reality as they advance through their days but they are just part of that crowd watching false images appearing real on the wall of the cave. They are viewing an illusion. Life is so much more than they appreciate. They do not have to betray themselves by living under beliefs, values and assumptions that, deep within them, they know are not right for them. They do not have to live as others expect them to live. They do not have to bury their dreams and live lives of utter mediocrity and boredom. They can break their chains, stand up for their biggest lives and see the world through a new set of eyes, eyes that see the truth rather than eyes that see lies."

"So, can you remind me what Stage Three is called, Julian?" I asked as we left the hotel and got into a taxicab.

"Stage Three is called 'Awareness of Wonder and Possibility.' When a seeker on the path home, to his true self—to his destiny—leaves the lie of Stage One and makes the decision to commit to walking towards the life that was meant for him at The Choicepoint of Stage Two, he will inevitably reach Stage Three. This is the time he begins to see there is an entirely different world out there than he has ever known. This is an incredible place for a human being to arrive at. Just think about it. The seeker has left the shackles of the crowd and is doing things in a much more authentic way. The limits are off. *He's ready to play with possibility.* He is reflecting on the values, beliefs and behaviors that feel right to him, regardless of what others think. He is being true to himself. He is also going deeper into himself than ever before, looking at his fears, his attitudes and all the ways of conducting his life that those around him have taught him to believe are the ways to succeed in the world. It's a time of much change, for sure. But it's also a time of great excitement."

"How so?"

"Because he really is beginning to see the truth. He is beginning to appreciate that this world of ours is a miracle. It is a gorgeous universe of wonder and possibility. Yes, at this stage, the seeker is leaving 'the known,' the place where he has lived his life to date, and walking directly into the unknown, a place of uncertainty and mystery. And, of course, that will give rise to fear because human beings always feel fear when they leave their areas of comfort. But it is only within the realm of the unknown that new possibilities live. Nothing new lives within the realm of the known, because if it did, it wouldn't be new, would it?" asked Julian.

"I think I follow you," I replied, seeing where Julian was

going with this line of reasoning. "You are saying that it's only in these unknown, foreign places that the highest possibilities for my life live. Right?"

"Exactly. Columbus was the first European to see the New World because he was willing to leave the places that he knew and visit the places that scared him—new, uncharted lands. All discoveries and all innovation are the result of women and men who dare to try the unknown. You need to walk towards your fears and be willing to go to new places to grow as a person and to uncover the treasures that are awaiting you as a human being. To stay in the world you have always lived in is to stay small and timid."

"Got it," I said with satisfaction.

"So as the seeker on the path to enlightenment leaves the lie he's lived under and makes the primary choice to reclaim his authentic power and true life, the way he will see the world begins to shift. He really will see the world through a new set of eyes. He really will see an entirely new experience of reality begin to unfold. He will walk into a brave new world rich with wonder and new choices. I know this has already started to occur in your life, Dar. And as you continue to walk the conscious path you have chosen, even more of this will unfold for you."

"Could you give me some examples?"

"Sure. As you move into Stage Three, you will begin to feel feelings that you have never felt. Or, to be more accurate, you will begin to feel the feelings that you once felt as a little child but then repressed when the world around you taught you that it was not polite to sing too loudly or shine too brightly. You will begin to feel the kind of joy that brings tears to your eyes and the kind of gratitude for being alive on a sun-soaked day that makes your heart beat more strongly."

"Very cool,'" I said with excitement, eager to experience the wonders Julian was speaking of and knowing that some of these wonders had already begun to enter my life since his coaching began.

"You will experience your feelings at a whole new level—and I should mention that you will not only begin to feel the highs you have not felt in many years, but some of the lows," Julian said. "Yes, at this stage you will feel greater happiness and delight than you have in years. But you will also be able to access your well of pain. You will begin to know yourself more deeply than ever before because you are leaving the lie that your life once was and awakening to the truth. And the truth is that you have denied much of your sadness. As you have left the person that you once were—as you have left your original nature through the process of self-betrayal, a part of you has died. And that has hurt you. As you have left your authentic self and walked out into this world of ours, a world that is filled with fear rather than love, a great sadness grew within you. Not only that, but the world hurt you in various ways. People crushed your hopes. People stifled your spirit. People stepped on your dreams. They told you to act in ways that you knew were not right for you. They taught you to be afraid of things and to behave in ways that the biggest and best part of you knew were wrong. But you did it."

"To be loved and to fit into the crowd," I chimed in, remembering what Julian had taught me.

"Exactly. So you must process through this sadness. You must work through the hurts that you have been carrying and the ancient wounds that have been festering within the sub-conscious part of you. In doing so, the narrow band of feeling that leads most people to live gray and colorless lives begins to widen. As you feel more of the sadness and pain you have swal-lowed, you also become able to feel more of the joys and delights of life. You will begin to feel moved by a sunrise and delighted by a rainbow. You will detect that the world is a far more colorful and vital place than you once thought it to be. You will also begin to feel more love than you have felt in a long time. And this will not just be love for those around you but love for yourself."

"Incredible."

"At Stage Three, as you leave the illusion that your life has been and start seeing the world for what it really is—a place of astonishing beauty—the pace of synchronicity in your life will quicken, as well. You see, my friend, the more courage and conviction you show in living the life that the universe wants you to live, the more it will send you its blessings. It will give you its green lights. Things will happen that will blow your mind. People will show up in your life at perfect times, almost as if they are angels sent to help you get whatever it is you want. In some ways, you will almost feel that you are guided by a pair of invisible hands leading you to the beautiful life that once lived only in the realm of your imagination. Your dreams will begin to become your reality."

As the cab drove along the barren city streets, Julian reached into his robe and pulled out a piece of cloth. Before I could say a word, he reached over and gently draped it over my eyes.

"Julian, what's going on?" I said with a mixture of surprise and excitement. "I can't see a thing."

"Just relax, amigo. There's a point to this. You see, most people on the planet today are wearing a blindfold of sorts as they venture through their lives. They are in the dark, so to speak. They are in a state of total ignorance about the way the world truly works and the role they are meant to play within it. Essentially, most people—and I do not mean to show any disrespect to anyone, I'm just speaking some truth here—are living in a way that can only be described as 'unconsciously incompetent.'"

"What exactly do you mean by that, Julian?" I questioned as we continued our cab ride to an unknown destination.

"Well, in learning any skill—whether that is the skill of learning how to ride a bicycle or the skill of living a great life—there are four plateaus the learner must proceed through en route to a level of mastery. The initial plateau or phase is that of 'unconscious incompetence.' At this point, the student is not only incompetent but has absolutely no awareness as to why he is incompetent. In other words, at this phase, the student doesn't know what he does not know. So, using the bike example, the student cannot ride the bike and has no idea what knowledge he lacks to ride the bike. Sadly, many people live the best years of their lives at this level of the beginner."

"They go through life with a metaphorical blindfold on, being unconscious of who they truly are and how they were meant to live," I confirmed, keeping the blindfold on.

"Exactly. Such people make no time to reflect on how they are conducting themselves, the quality and nature of the choices they make and what needs to improve in order for them to live their biggest games as human beings on the playing field of life. Now, if there's a willingness to improve, some people rise to the second phase, which is known as 'conscious incompetence.' At this level, the learner is still incompetent with respect to the skill but at least he has become conscious of all he does not know and needs to learn. In the bike scenario, he still cannot ride it but he knows he must improve his balance, hold the handlebars in a certain way and use the pedals in a specific fashion in order to move the bike forward. Awareness is growing. And as awareness of what you don't know grows, new choices can be made. And new—and better—choices cause positive changes."

"What about a human being at the level of 'conscious incompetence' with respect to the skill of living a life? What would that look like?"

"Excellent question," Julian noted as the cab sped up. "Such an individual would still be far from a place of mastery, but at least would be waking up to reality in the sense that he would be acutely aware of all he did not know and needed to work on. Though he would still be incompetent at living life, he would possess the awareness required to see all the mistakes he was making. For example, he could see all the areas in his life where his fears were running him or all the times where he was out of integrity. He could see all the instances in which he is not being authentic or settling for mediocrity instead of magnificence. And since awareness precedes choice and since new choices create new changes in one's life, he would be making some giant steps forward. This kind of knowledge would then bring him to the third plateau, which is known as 'conscious competence.' At this level, the student has become competent. Yet he still must invest much energy in paying attention to what he is doing; he has not yet reached a level of mastery but there is no doubt he is doing well. In terms of the bicycle metaphor, the learner can now ride the bike nicely. But he still must be very conscious of how he holds the bars, the way he balances himself on his bicycle and the way he pushes the pedals."

"And what does someone at the phase of 'conscious competence' *in his or her life* look like?"

"They are doing well. They have accessed many of the natural laws that govern the world. They have left the lie that their lives once were and become acutely conscious of all their self-betrayal. They have left the crowd and are now living lives on their own terms, listening to the silent whispers of their hearts and heeding the suggestions of their consciences. But they still have to make their daily choices in a very conscious and deliberate way. They still must pay a lot of attention to everything they do. Many seekers on the path to their greatest lives reach this place and I should tell you, it's a wonderful place to get to. But, if you are willing and if you are devoted, you can get to an even higher level of operating and that's the plateau of 'unconscious competence.' At this lofty plane, the student reaches the level of true mastery of the skill being learned. At this plateau, the rider of the bike doesn't have to think about anything anymore. He just runs outside, hops on his bike and races down the street, paying far more attention to the wind on his face and the sunbeams on his back than on how he positions the handlebars. And someone living life at this level is fully engaged in the present moment. He would be masterful in the way he advances through his days. He would be infinitely wise and awakened. And this would be a beautiful thing," observed Julian as the taxicab screeched to a stop.

"We're here, my friend. Please leave your blindfold on until we get inside the building."

"Where are we?"

"One of the most important things you must do at Stage Three of The 7 Stages of Self-Awakening is release control. You must be willing to let go. *You must be willing to surrender all you have known and walk into a new reality*. Yes, this can be very challenging, but it will also be one of the best moves you will ever make, opening up a universe of possibilities and a whole host of precious gifts. The writer Marcel Proust said it well when he observed: 'Do not wait for life. Do not long for it. Be aware, always and at every moment, that the miracle is in the here and now.' E. E. Cummings said it even more succinctly: 'It takes courage to grow up and become who you truly are.'"

We stepped out of the car and Julian led me by the arm to a building, the blindfold still covering my eyes.

"Okay, amigo, you can come out of the darkness now and into the place of wonder."

I took off the blindfold. I immediately realized that we were in one of the main exhibit halls of our local art gallery. Julian was grinning.

"All month long, the gallery is host to an international Salvador Dali exposition. They have some of his most famous work here. His art is incredible—I've spent hours each day here, just staring at his paintings. I brought you here to make a point that's relevant to Stage Three of the seeker's journey. Once you leave the lie that your life once was and have made the choice to awaken and walk the conscious path, Stage Three will inevitably occur in your life and you will begin to see the world through a new set of eyes, as I've suggested. This path will not always be an easy one to travel—you know that now. But it's the only path to walk if you want to live the noble life that was laid out for you. 'Everyday courage has few witnesses. But yours is no less noble because no drum beats before you and no crowds shout your name,' wrote Robert Louis Stevenson. The blindfold that once blocked you from seeing how big, beautiful and rich this world of ours truly is will come down and you will see your life as a work of art. Salvador Dali's art is like that of no other painter. He saw the world through a different set of lenses and, as a result, he created pieces that are breathtaking in their power and unrivaled in their creative impact. I want you to keep stepping out of the darkness that your life once was. I want you to keep being 'consciously competent' in the way you run your days so that one day, you will reach that level of mastery and authentic power known as 'unconscious competence.' I want you to create a life that, indeed, will be considered a work of art. You have that potential. We all do, as a matter of fact. It all comes down to whether you want to do the inner work required to get there. Become the Salvador Dali of your life, my friend, and just watch the wonders unfold."

The rest of the morning, Julian and I strolled through the gallery, studying the art and enjoying each other's company. Julian opened up even more to me, telling me about the personal challenges he had faced as a lawyer and some of the circumstances that led to him leaving the law and trekking to India in search of answers to the questions he had been struggling with. He made me laugh more than I had laughed in a long time as he shared some of his war stories and adventures as a jet-setting litigator. And he moved me to tears as he shared how his widely publicized demise as a lawyer had been prompted by the little-known death of his only child after a drunk driver collided with the car in which she had been a passenger.

"'Life will bring you pain all by itself,' Julian said, quoting the famed psychologist Milton Erickson, 'your responsibility is to create joy.' Life has handed me some pretty large setbacks. But I'm a survivor and nothing can keep me down. I've also discovered that nothing that happens to us in life has any meaning other than the meaning we attach to it. Pain and suffering only come from judgment. As we release judgment and stop labeling things as 'positive' or 'negative' and simply accept them as opportunities to evolve into our biggest selves, our lives transform. There really is no such thing as a 'bad experience' or even a good one. *Life just is*, if you get what I'm saying. Through the way we interpret and process the experiences of our lives, we shape our reality. Our thoughts form our world, in so many ways. I see life as a splendid adventure. The hard times fuel my growth and make me wiser. The easy straights fill me with joy and seem to be rewards for living in alignment with the natural rules of the game. As Peter told us last week, life really is short, my friend, and we need to take daily steps to access the greatness that resides within. Life is a sensational voyage and I, for one, intend to enjoy it."

# CHAPTER 7

# The Seeker Receives Instruction from Masters

*First say to yourself what you would be; and then do what you have to do.*

—Epictetus

*What if I should discover that the poorest of the beggars and the most impudent of offenders are all within me, and that I stand in need of the alms of my own kindness; that I myself am the enemy who must be loved—what then?*

—Carl Jung

It had been a full month since my last encounter with Julian at the art gallery. I had been getting up early each morning and spending much time in silent reflection, going deeper within myself than I had ever gone. I became intimately aware of many of the patterns I had been running over the years, ways of thinking, feeling and acting that, prior to my coaching with Julian, I had never recognized. Awareness really did precede new choices. How could I choose better ways to live if I wasn't even aware of what needed to be improved? And my new choices really did lead to new change. I began to see how often I'd sabotage myself and limit the size of the life I was living. I went behind my behaviors, and for the first time in my life, did some serious self-examination as to what the root causes of them were. It was a tremendously exciting time for me as I grew to know myself. It was also a time of some melancholy as I began to observe how frequently I betrayed myself.

During the weeks I was apart from Julian, I also started to catch myself just as I was about to fall into one of those old self-defeating behaviors I could now see had led me into so much pain and suffering. Whereas, in the past I would have reacted in a negative way, without thinking, I now would pause before I reacted. It was hard to believe how often people or circumstances would push my buttons. In the old days, I'd blame my feelings and reactions on the people or circumstances. Now, thanks to Julian's sage counsel, I took ownership over the way I felt and realized *it all began with me*. This was an amazing thing for me to observe and it made me feel much better about myself. I guess I truly was growing and becoming more of the person I was destined to be.

In a phone call I made to Julian, he confirmed this was, indeed, one of the most noticeable signs of personal growth. He also let me know that neuroscientists had recently discovered that human beings have a .25 second window of opportunity between a stimulus and the corresponding response to catch their thinking and make a better choice. He suggested that it was within this .25 second space that I could rescript much of my behavior and reshape much of my life, making the higher decisions required to lead me to a far more awakened state.

The more I thought about all that Julian had shared with me, the more I began to understand that he had developed a profoundly wise yet extraordinarily practical philosophy for the conduct of a beautiful life. Yes, my daily choices would have a big impact on the way my life turned out. I had a huge role in creating what I wanted. But the way in which my destiny would ultimately unfold would be the result of so much more than what I, as a human being, could choose or control. As Julian often told me in our coaching sessions: "You do your best and then let nature do the rest." All I could do was to try to be the best person I could become and live as truly as I possibly could at every stage of the path. Life would then take over and lead me to where I was meant to be. I might not always like where I ended up but Julian emphasized that I needed to trust that wherever I was guided was the place I would experience the greatest growth, the highest healing and the most effective learning. There was a higher order ultimately running the show, a higher order that was not possible for me to understand under the limited perception available to me as a human being.

I used to play a lot of tennis while I was growing up and Julian's personal philosophy about the partnership between fate and choice, as they impact on the way our destinies unfold, sometimes reminded me of that game. It seemed that the only thing I could control was what happened on my side of the court. My only obligation was to deliver my best serve, and hit my best shot. I had a duty, in respect to life, to let my light shine and take action around my dreams. To do anything less was to dishonor the gifts that had been granted to me. But once I did that, and the ball went onto the other side of the court, I needed to detach from outcomes—and relax. I needed to trust in the friendliness of this infinitely wise universe of ours. It was only my fear that caused me to worry about the results. Once I let go of the fear, Julian promised, and trusted in the larger plan, I would see that *things always worked out for the best.*

I also deepened my understanding of the imperative of personal responsibility and the notion of accountability in the month since Julian and I last met. While I did appreciate that fate had a rough destiny mapped out for me, I felt more clear than ever about the power I possessed to fill in the blanks as to how my destiny would look by the way I showed up in the moments of my days. If I was authentic, did what was right, applied my talents to create what I wanted and chased my dreams, there was no question in my mind that my life would work better than it ever had. "Heaven helps those who help themselves," Julian had told me. "You really can create much of your luck." It really was all one giant balancing act, between the power of my choices and the hands of fate, of making things happen and letting things happen, of doing and being.

Of all my new learning, perhaps what struck me most powerfully was the growing awareness of all that I had been resisting in my life. Julian was a strong believer in "constantly confronting one's resistances" and the more I considered this, the more I saw all the things I had been running from. The author Sam Keen once wrote that "we are caught by what we are running from." Truthful words.

Julian had requested that I meet him at a schoolhouse owned by the Stone Institute for Gifted Children. He had appointed a meeting time quite late in the evening and I wondered what my adventurous coach had planned for me during this learning session. I also wondered how much longer I would have the privilege of being coached by Julian. The media had not become aware that Julian was back in the city and I knew that he had been keeping a low profile. From what I could gather, he spent his days volunteering at the hospital where I'd met Peter, communing with Salvador Dali at the art gallery, working with me when the time was right and working on himself through meditation, reading, journaling and patient reflection. He also informed me that he spent a lot of time walking in the woods and communing with nature. Julian truly was a man of great simplicity. It was also becoming clear to me that Julian was a truly great man—period.

As I entered the building, I saw a piece of paper, with Julian's handwriting on it, taped to the wall. He had written: "Life is a growth school, ideally created to give us opportunities to learn each of the lessons we need to learn over the course of our lives on the planet. We live on 'Schoolhouse Earth.' And one of your teachers is enthusiastically awaiting your arrival. I'm in room 101. Tonight's program is entitled *Awakening Best Self*." At the bottom of the page were the following letters: "T.M.W.S.H.F." I knew this stood for The Monk Who Sold His Ferrari. Next to the letters was a smiley face.

I walked down the darkened hallway. Suddenly, I heard the sound of a drum beating. As I walked towards it, it became clear that it was emerging from Room 101. I had no idea what to expect next. The door was shut and the drum beats grew louder as I approached. My heart started to pound with a nervous excitement. What was happening on the other side of the door?

"Visit the places that frighten you" was one of the phrases I had committed to live by, based on Julian's teachings. So I bravely opened the door and walked in. The room was dark except for the luminous glow from hundreds of tiny candles placed in a large circle. In the center of the circle stood none other than Julian, wearing his robe and playing his drum in a rhythmic and dramatic fashion. His eyes were closed and he was softly chanting the following slogan: "Within your heart, all answers lie. Walk towards your fears and then you'll learn to fly." He kept repeating this over and over. Not once did he open his eyes. It was almost as if he was in a deep trance. I shut the door behind me and simply stood there. After about five minutes, Julian stopped beating the drum. The room was completely silent. He opened his eyes.

"Welcome, Dar. Forgive my unorthodox teaching methods," he said with a grin. "As always, judge by results. You will discover, as time passes, that my coaching process will work wonders in your life. Just keep trusting. You've been a brilliant student to date. I want to recognize you for that. And I know you are already drawing your biggest life towards you."

"Where do you want me to sit, Julian?" I asked, in a state of high anticipation for the life coaching I was about to receive.

"Come here, into the center of the Truth Circle. The Native American Indians believe that life is lived in a circle; 'The Circle of Life,' they call it. At the end of our lives, we return to the place where we first began the journey. A circle speaks of wholeness and integrity. Within this circle tonight, we will only speak the truth. *Remember, the purpose of life is all about making the journey home to wholeness, back to a place of integrity, back to your authentic self—the one that is fearless, all-knowing and of boundless love. The purpose of life is to close The Integrity Gap."*

"I'm not familiar with the concept of The Integrity Gap. Should I be?"

"No, amigo. I'm just introducing it to you now because you are ready for it. I've spoken since we first met about what happens to a human being after we are born—the process by which we lose the connection with who we truly are. We are born authentic and pure. We are born fearless and with wide-open hearts. We are born knowing the natural laws that rule the world and why we are here. But—and I know you now know this—we want to please those around us and fit into the crowd..."

"The crowd watching a figment of reality dancing on the cave wall rather than an accurate representation of the truth," I interjected, referring to the cave metaphor from Plato's *Republic* that Julian shared with me during the coaching session at the Camden Caves.

"Right on," he bellowed, pumping a fist into the air. "The process by which we leave our authentic self and become people that we are not—by taking on beliefs, values and behaviors from those around us—is known as *enculturation*. And as we leave our true selves, morphing into our social selves, a gap begins to form. We leave our original nature and assume the false mask of personality. We fall out of integrity, hence, The Integrity Gap. The greater the gap between who we truly are and the public personas that we present to the world, the less our lives will work. The greater the chasm, the less the universe will support us because we have forgotten who we are and are no longer playing by the rules we were meant to play by. With a wide Integrity Gap, we will feel little joy, have little energy and live small lives. We will be living in the 'cult of personality,' which is not the way we were meant to live. Your personality is not real. It is simply something you have created to be liked—no, to be loved. You have put on a social mask, out of fear."

"Seriously?"

"Seriously. A small child who craves love is running the show for most people. This little child is afraid of not being loved. This little child is afraid of not fitting in. This little child is projecting his mom and dad on all those other adults around him and hoping that if he acts like them—like the crowd—he will find the approval he so desperately seeks. Are you beginning to see why so many among us are afraid to walk this path of truth? At a very deep and often unnoticed level, they are afraid they will not be loved. And every human being has a primary desire to be cherished. So we fall into a trap. We betray ourselves, give up on our dreams and adopt ways of being that were never intended for us."

"And this sets up an Integrity Gap that shuts us down and limits our lives. And it's all driven by fear. I now see why it's so important for a person to work on himself. Once we do the inner work required to move through the fears that are running us, we move these shadows into the light of human awareness. And as you mentioned, moving a shadow into the light causes it to disappear. The fear leaves us."

"Actually, Dar, the fear not only begins to disappear, it becomes replaced by love. Like I told you, darkness is nothing more than an absence of light: once you pour the light of human awareness and understanding into the darkest recesses of your being, you will become a being filled with light. Where there was once fear, there will be love. Remember what it means to be 'en-light-ened': one filled with light. Every step you take to close The Integrity Gap is a step home, towards the state of enlightenment that you truly are. Every move you can make to be love when fear wants to own you, you reclaim—and remember—your original nature. Every single thing you do to present your biggest self to the world has the corresponding effect of helping you take back more of the authentic power that you were born with. That's why I told you I think the whole notion of self-improvement is nonsense. The job of every human being is not to improve—we already are perfection, at the deepest level, and you cannot improve upon perfection. Have I shared the story of the golden Buddha with you, amigo?"

"No, I don't believe you have."

Julian sat down in the center of the Truth Circle and crossed his legs. The room looked mystical as the candle flames flickered. Julian looked enormously peaceful and his gaze seemed to connect with a deep part of me. It almost felt as though he was looking inside me, calling for the most noble and real part of me to reveal itself.

"Many years ago, in the East, there was a band of monks who had a huge golden Buddha statue that they idolized. They would pray to it, meditate around it and cherish its presence in their lives. A time came when the place where they lived faced the threat of attack from foreign invaders. Each of the monks feared that they would lose the prized possession of their community, so they all began to think of ways to protect it. One of the monks came up with a simple yet seemingly effective plan: the monks would work together to place layers of mud over the golden Buddha in an attempt to cover it up and hide it. And the plan worked: the invaders did not find it."

"Very interesting."

"But there's more, my friend. Years later, a young monk was taking his morning walk when he saw something shimmering amidst the mountain dirt he had passed by so many times before. He called out to his monk sisters and brothers and they began to peel through the layers. And as they moved through each layer of mud covering up the golden Buddha, more and more gold began to show. Finally, with all the layers removed, the full glory of the golden Buddha could present itself. They beheld a priceless treasure."

"Great story," I acknowledged.

"Well, it serves as a powerful metaphor for us in this school-house tonight. You see, life is all about getting an education. Each day life will teach you the lessons you need to learn if you pay attention to it. The problem is that most people don't. The problem is that most people are asleep, unconscious. As you now know, they remain at Stage One of The 7 Stages of Self-Awakening. But as you awaken and move through the stages towards reclaiming your best self and the ultimate end-state of enlightenment, you will be getting to know your original nature. Each day will provide you with opportunities to move through another layer of the mud that is covering up the brilliance and gold that you truly are. And that's why the primary way to get back home and close The Integrity Gap is self-discovery and performing the inner work I often speak of. You must make the time to confront your resistances and examine yourself when frustrations or fears surface, rather than making it about others and avoiding self-responsibility. When you blame others for the things that anger or irritate you, you lose a precious chance to get to know more of the shadows that are running you. You lose the opportunity to go deep and bring what was within the realm of the subconscious into the realm of the conscious, where it can be healed and released. Every person alive today has layers of mud covering up our authentic selves. Some of us have more layers to move through than others. We assume these layers as we leave our authentic selves and join the crowd."

"And this process is known as enculturation," I added.

"Correct. The purpose of life is to remove the layers so more of the gold within us can shine and see the light of day, just as more of the golden Buddha peeked out as the monks removed the layers. And the exciting thing is that *every act of courage, every act of goodness and every act of self-responsibility will have an immediate payoff for you: each time you do what you know is the right thing and follow your truth rather than the dictates of the crowd, a little more of the mud covering up who you truly are begins to shine. Each time you act with love rather than fear, you become more of who you were meant to be. Every time you reach for your dreams and listen to your heart, you remember a little bit more of who you are.* This is how you get to know yourself. This is how you play your highest game. This is how you live your destiny."

Julian paused. "So what I must teach you today—the most important lesson you can learn on Schoolhouse Earth—is that *the purpose of life is to close The Integrity Gap.* Ideally, there would be no gap and the person that you present to the world would be the person you truly are. Ideally, the person you present to the world would be a perfect reflection of your authentic self. You would have no fear requiring you to pretend, in an effort to fit in and be loved. You would have so much self-love that it would not matter what others thought of you. So long as you were true to yourself, all would be good. And that, my friend, is what real success as a human being is all about."

"Your philosophy is profound, Julian. Life-altering, in fact. What are some of the specific tools I should be using here on 'Schoolhouse Earth,' as you call it, to close The Integrity Gap?"

"Writing in a journal on a regular basis is very powerful. This helps you get to know yourself and deepen your self-relationship. Your journal should be a place you visit and examine yourself. With the awareness that brings, you can then pledge to make better choices. I've also mentioned meditation and silence. Spending time alone in silence every day is a tool that will help you awaken and reclaim your authentic power. Of course, to succeed on Schoolhouse Earth, you will also need to have good teachers. And that brings me elegantly to Stage Four of The 7 Stages of Self-Awakening.

"Seekers on the path of awakening are like travelers leaving an old world and entering a new one. When you visit a new place, you need guides to give you direction and show you the way. Stage Four is about seeking 'Instruction from Masters.' At this stage, seekers turn to teachers, books and other types of learning resources. It is at Stage Four that many seekers journal for hours at a time and read book after book after book. Sometimes, a feeling of panic might even arise within you. You feel *frustrated* and afraid because your world is changing. There is so much to learn in so little time. Everything is in transition. By learning from many different sources you are playing the role of a good student. And you are more committed than ever in your quest for the truth about how life works and your role within it."

"Julian, this is *exactly* what I've been experiencing. The more I've been releasing control and walking into the unknown places of my life, the more questions have been coming up for me. I wonder who I truly am. I wonder what my destiny is. I wonder what my deepest values truly are. I struggle with the assumptions that I've made about the way the world works and want to know the true laws of nature upon which the world has been built. I've also been wondering whether there's a God and why I've had to suffer as I have. And I want to know how my life will turn out and exactly what I need to do to live my best, most authentic life."

"All those struggles are good. The fact that you are asking those big questions means you are growing and awakening. You are leaving the crowd and becoming more conscious. And so you question everything. Great! Asking the right question is often ninety percent of finding the right answer. In doing so you are discovering *your* truth and *your* authentic life. And remember, questioning unlocks the knowing that already exists within your heart. Ask the right question and I promise you, the answer you seek will surface—when the time is right."

"What do you mean by 'when the time is right,' Julian?"

"Well, one key natural law is this one: *we never get more than we can handle*. The path is lovingly planned for you and you will never, ever receive more knowledge or truth than you are ready for. So all the pieces come to you only when you are ready to receive them. The student must be patient. But the answers *will* come."

Julian continued: "Trust that you are exactly where you need to be. You are on the path that has been walked by many wise souls before you. Your experience is not unique. Just keep the faith and continue choosing to go deeper and deeper within yourself. All of the answers that you are looking for are within you. Yes, the books and teachers and seminars will help you. But remember one thing: reading the book of another person is a reflection of *their* truth. Hearing a speaker at a seminar means that you will hear *their* truth and *their* philosophy on the world and on life itself. That's fine at this stage of your journey. *Learning what others think will help you to figure out what you really think.* But don't make the mistake of believing that the truth of another person is necessarily your own truth. Don't be too much of a follower. Be a leader. Leaders go where no one has gone and blaze their *own* path. This whole adventure is about being authentic. As you move to higher and higher stages on the path to self-mastery, you will develop your *own* philosophy about the way life works and your place within it. You will select the truths of others that resonate with the deepest part of you. You will integrate the wisdom of others that rings true to you. And you must discard those ideas that do not speak to you and fail to make sense. In doing so, you will forge your own authentic code and constitution for living your biggest life. That's my definition of success—living your life in your own way. And authentic success is also about being in the process, in every moment of your days, of creating the life that you choose. You will not be living the life others have prescribed for you but living according to your heart's truth. And in so doing, you will grow into a power that will make you a force of nature in the world."

"This is truly fascinating, Julian. As I say, that's exactly what I'm going through right now. I've had this hunger within me awakened. I've let go of control more than ever before and am keenly aware of my ignorance. And the result is that I'm reading book after book. I'm searching for all these answers. I guess I really *have* become a seeker."

"Yes, Dar. You *are* becoming conscious. You *are* awakening. You are looking for ways to get back home. Some books preach the route to enlightenment or, at least, a happy life through positive thinking. Other books tell you to get out of your head and live in your heart. Yet other guides encourage you to become a 'go-getter,' set hundreds of goals, and chase after what you want. And other books invite you to 'be in the now' and let life gently show you what it has in store for you."

"Exactly. Who should I believe? Everything seems so contradictory. Do I live in the world or choose the spiritual path?"

"Ah," sighed Julian. "These are the questions that must be asked to find *your* truth. You really are growing and all this is good. You are seeking ways to close The Integrity Gap, to reclaim who you truly are and *remember* your authentic self. So you experiment with many different modalities and are open to many different teachers and this is perfect," noted Julian with a confident smile.

"There seems to be so much coming up. I'm starting to notice how far out of integrity I am—my Integrity Gap must be pretty large. I seem to wear my social mask in every possible instance. I think I've lived much of my life simply pleasing other people, my parents and others around me. I don't think I even know who I am anymore. You talk about having a great self-relationship and 'knowing thyself' as a means to enlightenment. I really have no idea who I am. That fills me with a great amount of sadness, to be honest." Tears began to well up in my eyes. I'd never felt such emotion.

"Feel that sadness, Dar. I've mentioned that to you before," replied Julian as he gently placed a hand on my shoulder.

"The more you can feel your feelings, the more they will complete themselves within you. Feelings are like rainstorms: they have a beginning, middle and an end. And as you complete each one of your feelings—whether those feelings are of anger, sadness, resentment or disappointment—you will move through the layers to remember the golden Buddha within you."

Julian patiently waited until I had regained my composure.

"Okay, Dar. If the *purpose* of life is to close The Integrity Gap, the question becomes what is the *process* by which life nudges you to do so. You see, as I've said, the universe wants you to win. Life is set up in such a way that you are hardwired to be happy and designed to be great."

"But I need to play by the rules of the game," I replied. "And if I'm asleep to them—still at Stage One—there's no way my life will work."

"Superb," exclaimed Julian as he gave me a hug. He began to beat the drum again, first softly—then lovingly. I knew this was his way of honoring me for the wisdom I was assimilating. Julian stopped and the room fell silent once again.

"The *process* by which nature or the universe or God or Infinite Intelligence—whatever label you want to put on the source of all creation—prods you to close your Integrity Gap is known as 'recycling.' Recycling is a term that explains how much of life works. Essentially it describes the phenomenon whereby, as we advance through life, we will be sent specific people and circumstances to teach us the lessons we most need to learn at that stage of the path. Let's say the lesson we need to get at a particular point of our journey is that of forgiveness. Well, in that case, this perfectly designed universe of ours will send us a person, for example, who betrays us. As always, we have a choice as to how we respond to whatever occurs in our lives. If we make it all about that other person and play the blame game, similar types of 'teachers' will show up in our lives. Similar types of people will *recycle*. The only problem is that the more you resist the designated lesson, the stronger, more intense and more painfully it will revisit you."

"So it will get my attention, right?"

"Yes. Just remember, what you resist will persist but what you befriend, you will eventually transcend. Nature wants you to close The Integrity Gap, learn your lessons while you walk Schoolhouse Earth and, in so doing, get home to your place of authenticity. Recycling occurs to support this movement, this journey to awaken your best self. But if you are asleep to the process of how life works, life will hit you harder. If you pay attention and wake up and live a *conscious* life by assuming personal responsibility for your healing and growth, you will learn the designated lesson and move closer to your true self. As you accept—instead of resist—your lessons and learning, the gap will close and life will get better."

"Incredible," was the only reply that came to mind on hearing Julian's understanding of how life works. I realized that if I blamed others for what provoked anger or irritation or jealousy within me, I was resisting an opportunity to learn a lesson intended for me. The lesson would recur in my life, with greater intensity and suffering. To me, the essential point was simply this: *by taking personal responsibility for what went on within me and by getting to know myself and the root causes of my negative reactions, I could literally minimize recycling in my life.* By refusing to blame others for my less than loving responses, I could dramatically cut down on the hurts of life. I'd be playing by the laws of nature so nature would support me. I'd be awake to *the truth* of the way life really works so life would hand me greater rewards.

Julian stood up and left the Truth Circle, walking over to a blackboard on the other side of the classroom. He had placed a series of candles next to the blackboard so I could see what he drew on it. He used the chalk to make a large circle. He divided it into quadrants. In the first quadrant he wrote "Mind." In the second he wrote "Body." In the third he wrote "Emotions." And in the fourth he wrote the word "Spirit." Above the circle he wrote the following words: "The 4 Awakenings." He looked at me and continued his discourse.

"As I mentioned to you, taking the leader's journey back home to your authentic self—and this is a *leadership* journey—is all about closing The Integrity Gap. Integrity means wholeness. Wholeness is reflected by a circle. The *purpose* of life is to return to wholeness. The *process* by which life supports that return is called recycling. The final piece involves the specific *practices* that close The Integrity Gap. At the instruction stage of the path to awakening—Stage Four—you begin to make conscious choices to get back to wholeness. There are four dimensions of your authentic self that need to be awakened for you to become whole once again. When you awaken these four dimensions, you will remember who you truly are. So here are The 4 Awakenings," Julian said, pointing to the board. "As you journey home, you must awaken your mind *and* your body *and* your emotions *and* your spirit."

"This is very interesting, Julian. I've been struggling with this point. Some books, as you mentioned, say that we find our best lives when we cultivate the highest potential of our minds. These authors suggest that we should read more books and learn more to keep exploring the quality of our thinking. They say our thoughts create reality. They say that our lives will transform when we change what we think."

"That's quite true, Dar. But that's not the end of the story. Awakening the mind is only *twenty-five percent* of getting back to wholeness and restoring your integrity. Yes, you must awaken the mind, which means exploring your core beliefs, your assumptions and your fears. This can be done by learning and discovering the truths of other people through their books, CDs and seminars. Awakening the mind—what I refer to as The First Awakening—can also be done by journaling, patient reflection and by being silent so that you pay more attention to the way that you live and become aware of all that you do not know. The First Awakening is all about accumulation, knowledge, learning and being conscious of the higher choices available to you. This is the intellectual work that needs to be done by a student on the spiritual path. But along with awakening the mind there are three other dimensions to be awakened to return to wholeness and close any Integrity Gap: the body, the emotions and the spirit. You must awaken the body, for sure. A healthy mind without a healthy body reflects no integrity. There's no wholeness there. So along with The First Awakening, you must perform The Second Awakening as well."

"So what can I do to awaken my body?"

"Regular exercise, a superb diet, sunlight, massage, fresh air, plenty of water, vitamins and supplements, reiki, yoga . . ."

"I get the point, Julian," I responded. "There are a whole series of tools that are available to me, aren't there?"

"Absolutely. The Second Awakening—the healing of the body—is all about making sure that your physical dimension is in wonderful condition. And *while* you awaken the mind along with the body, make sure you awaken your emotions. This is the Third Awakening. It is important that you process through any anger that you have been carrying through life. It's important that you forgive any people who have wounded and hurt you. Forgiveness is something you do for yourself, you know?"

"I didn't know that," I offered sincerely.

"It is. When you have not forgiven someone, it is almost as if you are carrying that person on your back—which is a very heavy load. And once you forgive them, you release them. You can finally move on with life. They are no longer pulling you down and you are much more free as a human being. But I must tell you that forgiving someone is different from condoning his or her behavior. Forgiving them is simply seeing that people in pain do painful things, as I said earlier."

"But is it really healthy not to speak out against hurtful behavior?" I asked.

"I guess what I'm trying to tell you is that one must go deeper and realize the truth beneath your judgment about other people. I encourage you to understand that people who hurt other people have themselves been hurt. People who do not love themselves cannot show love to others. *And people who do not have any self-respect have no idea how to give respect to others.* Keep on remembering this and you will be set free. Keep on journaling about these realities and timeless truths so that they sink deeper within your consciousness. Keep on putting a voice to your fears and they will move through you. Remember, feelings are like rainstorms, with a beginning, a middle and an end. If we stifle them, they will fester like wounds. If we pay attention to them and bring them into the light of our awareness, we will move through them and they will complete. And we will move to greater and greater health."

"And what about The Fourth Awakening, that of the spirit?" I asked as I walked over to the chalkboard and pointed to the final quadrant.

"Excellent question. When we awaken the spirit we nurture our highest self. This looks like different things to different people. To some, the spirit may involve prayer or talking to God. For others, caring for the spirit may be reflected by communing with nature or listening to moving music. For yet others, awakening the spirit involves service, volunteerism, and living for a crusade larger than oneself. Whatever modality or tools that you use, just remember that we need to begin the process of awakening *all four of our core dimensions at the same time.*"

"This seems like a lot of work, Julian," I stated honestly.

"Remember, the thousand-mile journey begins with a single step. You don't have to do all of this in a week or a month. Just make sure that every single day, you do *something* to awaken to who you truly are, no matter how insignificant it may appear to be. I deeply recommend that you make a commitment to yourself here in this room. Use much of the first sixty minutes of every day—your holy hour—to work on your Four Awakenings. This is an incredibly powerful way to live your biggest life and realize your destiny."

"I can do that," I pledged. "I've already been spending time each morning, as you told me to do, advancing my inner work. This makes so much sense, Julian."

"Make a self-promise here in this room that you will spend time at the beginning of your day working on the four core areas of your inner life. You might spend this time journaling or reading or meditating. You could use part of this time for prayer and another part of the hour for exercise. This one strategy alone really will transform your life if you adopt it and integrate it into your days. Trust me on this one. You see, my friend, if you do not act on life, life will act on you. The days will slip into weeks and the weeks into months . . . before you know it, your life will be over. Do not let the brilliant and beautiful treasure of your life slip away. Keep making choices that will help you remember who you are. Take sixty minutes at the beginning of your day to do the inner work required to deepen yourself and to awaken to the golden Buddha within you. It will be the single greatest gift you have ever given yourself."

Julian returned to the Truth Circle.

"There is one final piece around Stage Four—the stage of Instruction from Masters—that I want to share with you. It is a very wise philosophy to connect to your mortality every day. Remember that life is short and you don't know when it's going to end. We both could be taken tomorrow, Dar. The key is to play your highest game and to live your greatest possibility now. Wise people remind themselves that every day could be their last. In doing so, they make it their commitment to be love rather than fear during the hours of their day." Julian reached over to a desk next to him and lifted up an elegant piece of writing paper.

He continued. "We all have the choice and opportunity to write the story of our lives if we want to. Each day is an opportunity to make a difference in how our obituary will read. Life need not act on us. We can choose to take conscious steps within the hours of our days to close The Integrity Gap and reduce recycling. We can make a daily decision to do something to promote The Four Awakenings. We can use each day as a springboard to live a higher and bigger life. In our choices, our *specific* destiny is shaped."

"One of the most powerful things you can do is to write the story of your life in advance. It may not turn out exactly as you articulate it, but as the old saying goes: 'If you don't know where you're going, any road will get you there.' I'd rather have a plan in place than no plan at all. You know my philosophy: one should do one's best and then let nature do the rest. Try your best, set clear intentions, chase your dreams and then accept what comes. Life's a gentle balance between making things happen and *letting* things happen. Do the *very* best you know how to do. Set your goals and state your intentions, chase your dreams as to what you want to receive from life. Then have the bravery and wisdom to let go. Surrender your intentions and accept *whatever* comes, knowing that it is for the best, even if it may not seem like it at the time. Life is a beautiful tapestry that has been perfectly woven together. We often do not receive what we want but we *always* receive what we need. We always get what's in our highest interest. That's one of life's *greatest* lessons."

"So what do you want me to do?"

"I want you to write the story of your life. I want you to write your obituary. I want you to dream big again and play with the potential that your life is meant to be, my friend. This is an emotional experience; it may even bring tears to your eyes. But I want you to write with all your emotion and every ounce of your love. Open your heart to this exercise."

In that room, on that night in spring, I wrote the story of my life, surrounded by candles and a loving person who wanted the best for me. I wrote about the person I wanted to become and the life I wanted to create. I wrote about the woman I would find and the husband I would become. I wrote about the family life that I had always felt I deserved. And I wrote what I wanted my life to stand for as a human being. I wrote powerfully about the values, authentic beliefs and standards that I would hold myself to. I dedicated myself, on that magical evening, to playing my biggest game as a person and letting the light that I had discovered within myself see the light of day. The layers over my gold would come off. The chains that had bound me would continue to be broken. I would keep moving towards the truth and enlightenment. I would keep waking up to life.

Tears began to flow from my eyes. I began to cry out loud. Soon I was sobbing like a little child. Julian began to cry as well, clearly moved by my courage as well as by my willingness to "visit the places that frightened me" and go deeper than I'd ever gone. I could feel that this man's heart was wide open. He put his arms around me and comforted me. Then he asked my permission to read what I had written. I was happy to share the longings of my heart.

After he put down the paper he looked at me and simply said: "Beautiful. You're making your way back home."

# CHAPTER 8

# The Student Begins to Transform and Recreate Himself

*"A dreamer is one who can only find his way by moonlight, and his punishment is that he sees the dawn before the rest of the world."*

—Oscar Wilde

*Small doubt, small enlightenment. Great doubt, great enlightenment.*

—Zen saying

*In a dark time, the eye begins to see.*

—Theodore Roethke

This was the most difficult time of my life. It had been six weeks since I had met Julian at the schoolhouse. I now saw the world through a new set of eyes and the very foundations upon which my old world rested had begun to crumble. Much of the time, I wondered what was happening and sometimes felt confused. On leaving me at the end of our last session, Julian had explained to me that as I let go of my old way of seeing things, my *greatest* fears would surface and I would cling to what I once knew, my old world view. He said that, as always, I had choices around everything. I could continue to move farther along the path home towards who I truly was or I could resist this leadership journey and remain stagnant. Julian quoted the philosopher Joseph Campbell who said: "The heroic life is living the individual adventure. To refuse the call means stagnation." In the deepest place within me, I wanted to keep advancing along the journey I had begun when I first met Julian at the motivational seminar but, more and more, it became harder.

What if Julian was wrong, I sometimes wondered. What if the way he sees the world and all his theories were wrong? What if my old way of seeing the world was correct and letting go of this familiar paradigm was going to take me into an unknown place where my life could get even worse? What if all those beliefs and assumptions I'd relied on my whole life— such as, "If you give too much to others, they will take advantage of you," or "The only way to succeed is to dominate the competition" or "The more one accumulates, the happier one feels"—were the *real* truths that rule the world? If I didn't obey them, maybe my life would become a *total* failure. Maybe Julian—though well-meaning—was out of balance and extreme in his philosophy.

Much of my time at work was a blur. I was consumed by the internal struggle I was facing. In moments of clarity, I realized that perhaps my confusion arose from the fact that I had one foot remaining in my old world and one foot entering a whole new one. I had found a quotation from Aristotle that made some sense of the challenges I was encountering on this voyage home to authenticity and my greatest life. I placed it on my bathroom mirror so I could read it each morning. Here's what it said:

*The beauty of the soul shines out when a person bears with composure one mischance after another, not because he does not feel them, but because he is one of high and heroic temper.*

It was scary—letting go of the world I knew and opening up to a new one I'd never known. But Julian told me that we are most alive when we are walking into the unknown and have the courage to walk through our fear walls. I also kept on reminding myself about what Julian had taught me about confusion always giving way to clarity and chaos eventually resulting in confidence. I *had* to trust Julian. None of my friends would understand what I was talking about these days and my work colleagues would have thought I was going crazy. During this period, I felt very alone and decided to spend a lot of time in nature. I would go out and walk in the woods. I somehow felt comforted. I felt part of a larger universe and a sense of peace filled me.

During this period of intense self-examination and transition, I would wake up in the middle of the night, sweating and shaking, sometimes with a sharp pain searing my heart. "What did I get myself into with this coaching process?" I would wonder. Things were *so* much easier before. I can see why philosophers have said that ignorance is bliss. I may not have known the truth before I met Julian, but there was some comfort in the illusion of my old life.

And yet, along with all the giant fears and confusion that

had begun to present themselves and all the questions that raced through my mind and all the old pain that began to surface as I went deep into my worldview, came a new-found sense of joy. It didn't happen very often, at first, but I began to *feel* more alive than I'd ever felt in my lifetime. Maybe I really was awakening to life as never before. All this happened as I began to process through those "ancient wounds" Julian had spoken of, and take responsibility for the mistakes I had made in the past. By reflecting on my childhood as well as adult experiences, emotions and old, long-forgotten memories began to appear. I would journal about them on a daily basis. I also would write letters to myself as a way to process through the feelings. And the more I began to feel my feelings, the deeper I went within myself. It really was as if I was moving through different layers, peeling away at the old so I could get to the truth. I was getting to know who I truly was. And Julian said that was "noble work."

Again, I need to be honest with you: this process wasn't an easy one. But it became *extremely* fulfilling, the deeper I went. And as I say, more and more, I started feeling a happiness that I hadn't felt before. The place of knowing deep within me knew that this was *real* joy.

One morning I got up at the crack of dawn and watched the sun come up. I found myself crying, awestruck at the beauty of this natural scene from nature. At other times, the music that I used to listen to on a daily basis was now something that I felt at a whole new level. A smile would come to my face as I felt moved by a brilliantly written opera or inspired by a pop song. And the way I related to people also began to change. I saw my friends and family members as well as my colleagues through a new set of lenses and felt a love for them I'd never known. Things people did that would have irritated me in the past bothered me far less because I realized they were simply acting from their wounds and their fears. They were doing the best they could do based on what they knew, and as Maya Angelou has said: "When we know better, we can do better." I reminded myself that deep within each and every one of them, there lay gold, magnificence and a loving human being. Every time someone did something to hurt me, even in the smallest of ways, I remembered Julian's point that "people in pain do painful things." People in fear act in fearful ways. They needed my forgiveness, not my anger. If I could not find forgiveness within myself, I needed to take responsibility for that and go deeper until I could access more of my heart. Within every thing that bothered me about another person there lived a gift of personal growth. In every circumstance that caused me frustration, there lay a superb opportunity to move through one of my own layers and, in so doing, to *remember* more of my best self—to reclaim more of my authentic power. The choice was mine: *blame or reclaim.*

This was a new philosophy for me, to state the obvious. Few people from the world I came from thought this way. But it felt right; the place of knowing within me knew that the more I embraced this way of living, the better my life would become. My instincts told me this way to live was the way of wisdom.

Julian had asked me to meet him at the Metro Zoo. In particular, he had asked me to show up at the section known as

Butterfly Heaven, which was home to thousands of butterflies, from the purely domestic to the highly exotic.

As I made my way to the designated location, the smell of the sweet flowers that lined the walkway brought a wonderful feeling to me and reminded me of the beauty of life. Life truly is a lovely blessing. So often, we get wrapped up in what's not working within our lives and pay no attention to the things that are. Julian had told me that one of the natural laws that run the world is that *when you focus on what you don't want in your life, you actually block what you do want from entering*. And what you invest your attention in will grow in your life. Focus on what you don't want and you'll get more of it. The world is a mirror. As he taught me, we receive from life not what we want but who we are, as spiritual beings. I had come to realize that, in so many ways, the simple pleasures of life are the most fulfilling. So that's what I began to focus on.

I looked around for Julian, but he was nowhere to be found. I actually asked a few of the guides who were there to serve tourists whether they had seen a good-looking man wearing a monk's robe. "There's no way you could miss him," I said. They smiled and said they hadn't seen such a person. I used the opportunity, while waiting for Julian to arrive, to review some of the notes I had made in my journal. I found that the act of writing not only recorded the steps of this remarkable journey I had embarked upon but my journal offered me a vehicle to get to know myself, to try to gain clarity over the awakening that was occurring in my life.

Journaling allowed me to think on paper and then to step out of myself and objectively evaluate my thoughts and actions.

Journaling allowed me the chance to literally think about the quality of my thinking. If one way I thought or behaved was not well-suited to the life I was dedicated to creating, I could make new choices that were more aligned with who I wanted to become and what I wanted to have. It just felt great to be able to have a place for self-expression and, as Julian described it, a conversation with myself. The point was well taken: if we don't have conversations with ourselves, how can we get to know ourselves? And the deeper we know ourselves, the more we can make authentic choices to make the leadership journey back home to the place that we have always known, at our core, we have wanted to be. In the Greco-Roman temples of the past, above the entrance one would often find the following words: "Know thyself and you will know the universe and the gods." This made more sense to me than ever before.

I got up and continued looking for Julian, but after ten minutes or so, I still had seen no sign of him. All of a sudden, I heard a loud knock coming from one of the glass rooms where the rare butterflies were housed. I looked in and could not believe my eyes. Julian never ceased to amaze me! He was inside the enclosure, covered by hundreds of the most breathtakingly beautiful butterflies I had ever seen. There were so many colors and so much life in that room. He still had on his red robe. He still had on his ever-present sandals. But this time, Julian also had on one of those hats that zookeepers often wear, with a net that completely covered his face. He was laughing as he shouted to me through the glass: "Come on in here, amigo. Today's lesson is a big one! And I know you're ready to discover it. There's one of these hats for you outside the door; I've arranged everything with the zoo."

I made my way to the door and put on the hat with the net dangling from it, as instructed by my eccentric but highly effective life coach. I entered the room and was awestruck at the miracle of nature that those butterflies embodied. Maybe the world is perfect and everything that unfolds does so according to a vastly intelligent plan. We try to understand why our lives play out as they do, but perhaps we are trying to make sense of something that has been created by an intelligence higher than human reason. Perhaps there is a perfection to *each* of our lives, a perfection that we miss if we look through the lenses of judgment and fear. Yes, our choices count. Yes, actions have consequences. Yes, we have much power to sculpt the way our destinies look. But there is a much more powerful force that is ultimately at play and in control.

Julian looked like a little kid, playing with the butterflies, revealing a sense of wonder and joy. He was laughing and clapping his hands as he flitted around the room, butterflies in tow. He then waved the butterflies off; they seemed to do as he instructed. He walked towards me.

"How are you doing, my friend?" he asked happily as he walked over and embraced me, a few butterflies remaining perched on his shoulder.

"Well, I've had better weeks," I replied, speaking truthfully. "So much is coming up for me. I don't know whether I'm coming or going sometimes, Julian. There is actually a lot of pain that I'm experiencing. I never thought this path of awakening would involve suffering."

"It's all part of the seven-stage process, Dar. This path requires immense courage. You are learning that through first-hand experience, which is the best way to learn. No book could ever come close to teaching you what life itself can teach you if you live it with your eyes wide open and are awake to its lessons. To risk is to live, my friend. We play small, thinking that's a safe way to live when that's actually the most unsafe place to be. That's part of the illusion."

"I agree, Julian. Neale Donald Walsh said: 'You are so afraid to live, so afraid of life itself, that you've given up the very nature of your being in trade for security.'"

"Beautiful," said Julian. "Never heard that one." He closed his eyes, apparently in contemplation, absorbing what I'd just said. Julian was a great listener. I loved being with him. He made me feel special.

"Here, have a look at this," Julian said as he pointed to a cocoon. "Richard Bach once wrote that 'what the caterpillar sees as the end of the world the master sees as the butterfly.'"

Those words spoke to me at a soul level. They *felt* right.

Julian continued. "You are going through a metamorphosis. You are experiencing a deep transformation. You lived your entire life as one big lie. You betrayed yourself and lived inauthentically, simply to fit into the crowd. Your choices and conduct were based on an illusion. Remember those false images that appeared real on the wall of the cave?"

"How could I ever forget, Julian?" I replied.

"You'll recall that Stage Two of the truth-seeker's path involves a basic choice: to remain asleep and small or to embark on a conscious journey towards enlightenment and her biggest self. If the latter decision is made, the seeker then moves through Stage Three, where she sees a whole new reality beginning to unfold, and Stage Four, where she craves the answers offered by masters as to what's happening to her and seeks a truer understanding of the world that exists behind the illusion. That brings us to Stage Five, the stage of 'Transformation and Rebirth.' It's a hard, hard time for the seeker because it's a time of *deep* transition. It's also the most exciting and important time of her life. Growth sometimes comes in difficult ways. But growth is always good. 'The way to your dreams can only be found with one foot in eternity and the other on shaky ground,' is how noted thinker Rick Tarquinio puts it."

Julian continued: "I know how confused you must feel these days. I understand the pain that you are enduring. There *is* suffering involved as you walk the path. I do not want to minimize what you're going through. But I must tell you that, if you could look down at your life from a fifty-thousand-foot perspective, *everything* that's happening is very beautiful."

"Beautiful? I've never suffered so much in my life. I've never been so confused in my life. My life seems to be moving into chaos rather than getting to a better place."

"That's just your perception right now," replied Julian. "Your human eyes see confusion and chaos. But you are in the process of gaining new vision. As you do, you will see that all that is happening to you is part of the process of letting go of your old paradigm for living. All that is occurring for you is a reflection of the fact that you are going through a time of massive growth. You are releasing everything you know and all the ways of seeing and behaving that governed your former life. And as you let go and empty yourself of all that you have been, you are making room in your life for new things to enter. You are making space for a new consciousness and a new way of operating and being. Yes, it's messy at times. How could it not be? The very foundations upon which you have lived your life are being challenged and then torn down. But trust me when I say that this is the best thing that's ever happened to you. Your mind is awakening. Your heart is opening. Your emotions are healing and your spirit is soaring. You are reclaiming your authentic power, which is far different from the external power provided by big titles, large bank accounts and corner offices. Those things come and go with the tides of life. And when they are gone, so is your power. But no one can take authentic power away from you, Dar. You earn it and then you own it—forever. So all this *is* beautiful. You are letting go of the control that once dominated your days. Like a caterpillar going through a cocoon, you are moving through the darkness and becoming something new. And yes, it's dark in that cocoon and on some days it may seem that there's no way out. But, in truth, the caterpillar is becoming a butterfly. Stagnation is turning into freedom. This is what deep change looks like and I hear you when you say it's not pleasant. At this stage of your journey as a seeker, it's almost as if the entire inner government by which you previously ran your life is being toppled and replaced by a whole new regime. There's a revolution underway. New beliefs are forming. New assumptions in terms of the way the world works are being forged. Fears are being released and transcended. A greater commitment to personal authenticity is being realized. Do you see how incredible this is? Try not to resist what's going on. You are headed to a wonderful place, my friend. The transition phases of our lives are the richest times of life. You are walking towards the light. The darkness will pass. The butterfly is coming."

"Really?" I couldn't help but ask.

"The laws of nature explain the laws of life," offered Julian. "You know that. A caterpillar cannot remain in the cocoon forever. A butterfly *must* emerge *when the time is right*. Just trust in nature's timing; it's not on the same clock as you. Remember that always. Your pain will pass—it always does. And as Carl Jung said: 'There is no coming to consciousness without pain.' Again, release control and just realize that there is a larger unfolding taking place. And all good."

"How do you know this is true?"

"Because I've walked this path to awakening in my own life. Remember what T. S. Eliot said: 'Only those who will risk going too far can possibly find out how far one can go.' You are going through what the mystics have called the dark night of the soul. I know that you're questioning everything. That's good. Questioning everything means you are no longer taking the status quo as truth. You are no longer a sheep blindly following the flock. You are waking up and growing. That's what leaders do. They leave the crowd once and for all and create their own paths. Mahatma Gandhi didn't follow the crowd. He set his own original vision and then had courage to stand by it. Helen Keller, Amelia Earhart, Mother Teresa, Martin Luther King Jr. and all other leaders—from leaders of nations to leaders in the arts like Salvador Dali and Picasso—did the same thing. Dali didn't try to be more like Rembrandt or Michelangelo. He lived out of his own imagination and had the bravery to pour the creative brilliance that had been embedded in his heart out into the world."

"So true," I acknowledged, letting two butterflies rest on one of my hands.

"You are no longer living your life to please others and to fit in because you are afraid of being abandoned. Instead, you are moving into your heart and beginning to pour more love into the world by the way you show up fully as a human being. You really are reclaiming your authenticity. You are becoming a butterfly and regaining your freedom. I'm so happy for you. And yes, this process creates pain in one's life."

Julian continued with another helpful metaphor. "When a baby comes down the birth canal, there is tremendous pain involved. But the baby and the mother do not give up. They persist through the transition phase, knowing that the outcome will be a miracle. You *will* experience a miracle if you are willing and keep choosing. We always have choices, as human beings. Each of us has far more choices than we are aware of. We think we are so limited in life that we *have* to live and do what we currently do. That's just more of the language that victims are prone to use. It's *always* up to you—how far along the path home from your social self to your authentic self you want to go. Some people never get on the conscious path and stay asleep an entire lifetime. Others make some steps home and remember some of who they truly are. And a handful of women and men have made it all the way home and completely remember who they are. These courageous souls fully reclaimed their authentic power, a power that each of us has within us, and are known to the world as 'enlightened ones.' These were true leaders on the planet, the spiritual giants, if you will. The pain that you are now enduring is because you are coming down the birth canal. You are experiencing a rebirth and a whole new being will emerge when the time is right. This universe is far more intelligent than we give it credit for, it really is. There is a brilliant coherence that runs our lives. The more we can stop trying to force outcomes and simply be in the flow, the more the magic that our lives are meant to be will appear. Trying to make everything happen and force results without balancing things off with a willingness to let things happen is nothing more than control. Just become aware that you are going through a time of transformation and be in the moment with it. Make a decision to enjoy and appreciate what you are going through and where it is taking you. Simply experience it without labeling it as bad. Release all judgment—it's only a part of the illusion. It's not real. The crowd taught you this kind of thing is 'bad.' Have faith. Feel the feelings that are coming up and process through them to completion. In the passage of time, you will look back at this as *the defining moment* of your entire life."

Now Julian pulled a well-worn book from his knapsack. "Here, look at this," he said. "These are some of the poems of Rumi. I love them." He read from a page: *"I saw grief drinking a cup of sorrow and called out, 'It tastes sweet, does it not?' 'You've caught me,' grief answered, 'and you've ruined my business. How can I sell sorrow when you know it's a blessing?'* Your sorrow is, in truth, a blessing. It is shaping and awakening you. Please remember that as you go through the fifth stage."

"Well, how do I get through this stage, then, Julian? I have to be honest with you. I feel like giving up. I don't know who to listen to anymore. My friends and colleagues come from a different world. Part of me knows they belong to the crowd and their beliefs are based on an illusion. But it's *so* hard to disregard what they tell me. I guess what I'm saying is that it's hard, at times, to remember that the way I used to see the world is based upon a lie and that there's a whole new and far more truthful way of operating as a human being. I feel like I'm caught between two worlds. Sometimes, I find myself questioning whether everything you're saying to me is indeed the truth. I don't question your honesty and integrity at all. That's not what I'm saying, Julian. I'm just wondering—what if you're wrong? What if I'm just making my life worse and creating more complexity for myself?"

"Excellent work, Dar. The more you can put a voice to your fear, the more the fear will move through you. The more you can talk about this, the more the hidden shadows come out into the light where they can be examined and released. Thank you for speaking your truth; so few do. Remember, talking about your fear and bringing it out into the open is a lot like inviting the monster who lives in the basement upstairs to the kitchen table for a cup of tea. The monster starts to dissolve once it is brought into the light of your awareness. What was once hidden within the realm of the subconscious now enters the area of the conscious mind where you can examine and evaluate it, making choices around it if you wish to. Most fears are nothing more than an illusion. You know that now. And yet they rule our lives. They keep us small. They keep us chained and fill our lives with limitation rather than possibility. All I'm asking is that you keep on trusting me. *It's always darkest before dawn. A time comes in everyone's life when they have to play at the edges and take some big chances. A time comes for every seeker where he or she knows, deep down in the heart, that refusing to take the risk will resign them to a life of mediocrity. But making the leap, though it involves great fear along with great courage, will allow them to travel*

*to a whole new land. A land of potential, happiness and free-*
*dom. Go deep and listen to the inner voice within you. Then*
*trust in its guidance. 'Life shrinks or expands in proportion*
*to one's courage,' wrote Anais Nin."*

"You know what, Julian? I'm starting to hear some kind of
an inner voice getting louder within me these days. That's
another thing that's shifting. Before, I was simply being
guided by your wisdom. Your coaching is what led me to this
point. It's almost as if I couldn't access my inner wisdom and
my personal truth. But that's starting to change, now that I
think about it."

"So well said, Dar. And that's another reason why you want
to keep on having *conversations*, not only with yourself but
also with other people who are walking the same path you are
on. And many people in the world today are. As I mentioned to
you earlier, conversation deepens conviction. The more you
can converse about the things that you want to become, the
more you will be able to dedicate yourself to doing what needs
to be done."

Julian began to play with the butterflies. The child inside of
him was clearly alive and well. The butterflies seemed to love
him, resting on his arms and shoulders. I joined in. We looked
like two kids frolicking in a schoolyard, totally in the moment,
and fully alive, free of any self-consciousness or inhibition.
Maybe I had been taking life too seriously in the past. Maybe
this was the most important and rich time of my life. I knew
this was truth as I reflected more deeply. I felt it in my body,
at its very core. The chatter in my mind wanted to tell me otherwise. But Julian was right: often that chatter is nothing
more than the voice of fear. The head is a limiter, the heart the

liberator. More than ever, I wanted to play like a leader in my life. I wanted to show up fully and play big with my remaining days. I wanted to let go of my limitations and make the journey back home. I wanted to reclaim, remember and recover the person who I truly was, beneath all the layers that built up as I picked up the limiting beliefs, assumptions and fears of the world around me. My bigness *was* coming out.

We are literally afraid of who we truly are. We are afraid of our light. We are afraid of our brilliance. We are afraid of our highest possibility. We are afraid to stand tall and let our light shine into the world. With great gifts come great responsibility. My guess is that most human beings don't want to look at their gifts because they don't want to deal with the responsibility that those gifts present. The responsibility to live fearlessly and make a difference in the world. And in doing so, they shrink from their greatness. I vowed never to let that happen to me.

In the days that followed my meeting with Julian at the zoo, more and more pieces came to me. Things began to make so much sense. *Patience was required on this trek to truth and self-awakening.* If all that I wanted to know and occur in my life happened immediately, I guess there would be nothing left for the journey. The whole reason we are alive, I realized, is to spend our lives finding our way back home. And it is a *journey.* But many answers did start coming. I observed that they seemed to appear only when I was ready to accept them. Questions that I had been struggling with seemed to be answered in an almost organic way. The more inner work I did, the more solutions and growth I received. The deeper within myself I went, the more my outer world began to shift.

In my old world, I thought that the way to salvation and happiness was to focus on externals. In other words, I believed that a more expensive car or a hipper suit would make me feel better on the inside. But the more time I spent with Julian, the more I learned that happiness is an inside job. It's not about chasing greater net worth—it's about cultivating a greater self-worth. It's not about having more money but about finding more meaning. And it's not about only being successful but about being truly significant—a person who creates lasting value in the world. By this I mean everything seemed to unfold naturally. As if there was a higher intelligence leading me. I'd always fought life. I know that this was all about control. I now lived in a different way: I let life lead me. This is not to say that I didn't act in a responsible way. Everything in life *is* a delicate balance. I still set my goals, took the action I needed to take and acted in a practical way. But rather than resisting life, I relaxed. I surrendered more. *I did my best and let life do the rest.* If, after doing my best, something still didn't work out, I felt it wasn't meant to be. And something even more perfect for my personal evolution would present itself. When one door closes, another always opens and every ending truly is also a new beginning.

I began to balance making things happen with letting things happen. I began to balance doing with being. I began to balance using my mind with listening to my heart. Reason with passion. Ultimately, my guess is that I was beginning to balance Earth with Heaven.

# CHAPTER 9

# The Seeker Is Tested

*If there is something great in you, it will not appear
on your first call. It will not appear and come to you
easily, without any work and effort.*

—Ralph Waldo Emerson

In the four weeks since my visit with Julian at the zoo, so many
blessings had appeared in my life. My relationship with my
children, whom I saw every week, grew more open and loving.
I began to listen to them at a level never available to me in the
life I lived prior to meeting Julian, and the bonds of love
between us grew exponentially. They told me I was far more
relaxed, much more caring and so much more playful than
they had ever known me to be. I was finally growing into the
father I had always hoped to become.

As well, while attending a lecture on self-discovery and personal transformation one evening at our local library, I met
Sasha, a lovely and intelligent chiropractor. I fell in love with
her; I never thought I could feel that way about a woman. She
was so calm and grounded, so wise, loving and funny. I knew,
on meeting her, that we were destined to spend the rest of our

days together. It was just a feeling I had—one I intended to pay a lot of attention to as I went through my days.

Thanks to Julian's coaching as well as his "holy hour" concept, my inner world was recreated. To advance The First Awakening, I read many books to develop and refine my base of wisdom. I also journaled on a daily basis, refining the philosophy of life that I intended to follow. I had decided, thanks to Julian's advice, to do my own thinking rather than letting others do it for me. I flat out refused to live someone else's life— the life that the crowd encouraged me to live. But since awakening the mind is only twenty-five percent of what is required to return to wholeness and close The Integrity Gap, I also focused on nurturing the body, healing my emotions and caring for my spirit. Four times a week I would trek off to yoga class. Three times a week I set aside time to consider my emotional self and process through any repressed anger or latent sadness I had stored so that they did not subtly affect the way I thought, felt and behaved. And each day I would do something, no matter how small, to awaken my spiritual side. On some days I prayed. On others I would go and sit in the garden for part of my holy hour, just smelling the roses and feeling the rays of the sun on my face. And, of course, I always kept my commitment to remaining true to myself and living by the values that feel authentic to me rather than being pulled into the crowd at the forefront of my consciousness.

This all might seem as though I spent a lot of time and energy on awakening my biggest life. The truth of the matter is that the time I spent on my inner work was borrowed from all the time I would waste in my former incarnation, engaging in various distractions ranging from watching television to oversleeping. I also became clearer than ever that the reason I had spent so much time doing those things was that, at a deep and subconscious level, I was in pain. I was suffering from the fact that I had been betraying myself by not living the extraordinarily beautiful and full life I was destined to live. Until I began to know myself and increase my awareness of what was really going on within myself, I had no idea why I lived as I did. I just followed the crowd and didn't think much about it. I was caught up in the lie. I had been trapped within an illusion. And it was killing me. "How many people are trapped in their everyday habits: part numb, part frightened, part indifferent? To have a better life," said Albert Einstein, "we must keep choosing how we are living."

Life became a joy to live. I had more energy than I had ever felt. My friends all told me that I looked ten years younger. I felt so connected to other human beings. My confidence and desire to be a great human being exploded. And my business soared. I guess it's true what Julian so often told me: "We attract into our lives not what we want but who we are." As I become more loving, wise and authentic, this infinitely intelligent universe of ours reached out to me and offered me the wind beneath my wings.

Julian gave me his personal copy of *The Saint, The Surfer and The CEO*, the book I had noticed in his hotel room at The Q. A story written about a man on an odyssey to discover his greatest life, the book revolves around three special teachers who reveal powerful lessons that help him make his transformation. It was a wonderfully inspiring read and I loved the many quotations it contained. I can see why it spoke to Julian.

Near the end, one quotation in particular became a daily affir-mation for me during this time of my life. I posted it on to my bathroom mirror along with the Aristotle quotation I men-tioned earlier and read it aloud each morning. The words were from Henri Frederic Amiel and they were as follows:

*The process of life should be the birth of a soul.*
*This is the highest alchemy, and this justifies our*
*   presence on earth.*
*This is our calling and our virtue.*

Other books I read during that period that moved me to keep digging deep and shining more brightly in the world included *Hope for the Flowers* by Trina Paulus, *Siddharta* by Herman Hesse, *Synchronicity* by Joseph Jaworski, *Sacred Hoops* by Phil Jackson and a wonderful little book about never giving up called *The Go-Getter* by Peter B. Kyne. I had never fully appreciated the power of great books to introduce me to my best self.

At this time of great introspection and personal growth, I also devoted much time to fully understanding the process that Julian had been teaching me. I understood that The 7 Stages of Self-Awakening represented an elegant model of the path that every seeker has to travel to get home to her essen-tial self. It brought together so much of the thinking of many different cultures and of so many different mystics as to why we are here and the way our lives work in a simple, easily understandable structure. The journey Julian had described was the journey home to truth and enlightenment, two goals that human beings have reached for since the dawn of the species. I also understood that, while Julian was taking me through the process over a few months and setting up scenarios that would help me understand what each stage was about, I would *naturally* experience each and every one of the seven stages of the path as I moved through my life, so long as I remained willing and devoted to traveling this road to self-awakening and authenticity. As he once said, "The 7 Stages of Self-Awakening is the process that *every* seeker must walk as he heads home to the place where his heart has always wanted him to be." And rather than taking a few months, Julian explained that the journey could—in reality—take a lifetime to complete. As a matter of fact, not everyone who embarks on the path home will reach the destination. Most do not. But every single day offers us the opportunity to step a little closer to the ideal and become more of who we were meant to become. Every single day on the path brings greater blessings and more personal power. Every single moment on the conscious journey causes more of the layers covering the golden Buddha within us to shine through the mud of our fears, limiting beliefs and false assumptions. Julian had simply collapsed the process to help me understand it quickly. He was trying to offer me a clear and powerful framework explaining the spiritual path. He was trying to give me as much value as he could and help me as much as he could in the limited amount of time that he had.

I realized that there were so many people across the world that Julian wanted to serve and I knew he needed to get to his next assignment. I often expressed my gratitude to him for finding me and helping me transform my life, as he undoubtedly had. He had been a loyal friend to my father and I regularly told him so. This made him happy. "Friendship is an incredibly important thing to me, Dar. I value— and love—my friends. Your dad was a wonderful man. It is my joy to help you, in the only way I know how."

Recently, Julian had even told me that he wanted to get involved in the global peace movement and was exploring ways to be of service in that arena. Various political leaders were becoming aware of his work as his message spread and Julian mentioned that he welcomed the chance to help as much as he could. He felt strongly that his wisdom and philosophy could profoundly reduce conflict in many of the world's troubled spots such as the Middle East and Northern Ireland, just to name a few. I fully agreed and awaited the day that Julian emerged on the world stage as a statesman, showing presidents and prime ministers how opening their own hearts and reclaiming their best selves was the real key to ending wars, developing "win-win" alliances and making the world a better, more love-filled place. "To eliminate hatred in the world, we must first eliminate any hatred we carry within ourselves," Julian told me one evening as we chatted on the telephone. I knew he would have taken a bullet in defence of that truth.

Julian also shared with me that a film producer had somehow been able to find him a number of months ago. He was informed that there was much interest in a movie being made of his life and all he was doing to build a new world. Great things were unfolding for Julian. I knew he did not seek any attention and did what he did from the purest of intentions.

But I was happy to see Julian getting some of the recognition he deserved. He was an evangelist in the truest meaning of the word—he was all about spreading good news on a planet that desperately needs it.

I was to meet Julian at the courthouse at 9 A.M. He had informed me that he had planned a very special coaching session for me, one that would bring the next lesson to life in a way that was unforgettable.

As I walked up the concrete steps to the courthouse, a police officer rushed over to me. I was surprised when he knew my name.

"Mr. Sandersen?"

"Er, yes," I said, wondering what this was all about. "What's going on?"

"Just come with me, please. My name is Officer Perez and I've been asked to escort you into the building. I cannot say anything else—sworn to secrecy."

Part of me felt that Julian was behind this. But another part of me grew a little concerned. The police officer seemed so serious. Yet I was a decent, law-abiding citizen who minded his own business and kept out of trouble; what could the police want from me?

Officer Perez led me down a hallway lined with ancient paintings of judges in gowns and legal attire. He was completely silent and very official. I walked a step or two behind him. I had never been in the courthouse and was intrigued by the whole environment. I used to enjoy watching all the legal dramas that fill today's television screens. My mother had wanted me to become a lawyer.

"Here we are, Mr. Sandersen. Make it a great day, Sir," he said with a thin smile.

I had been delivered to Courtroom Number 6 and now stood before two huge wooden doors. The building smelled musty and the carpets were in dire need of replacement from many years of traffic. There was no one around. I pushed the doors open and entered the room, with no idea what to expect. My heart was beating rapidly.

The courtroom was empty except for two people. At the front of the cavernous space was an elderly judge who sat behind the bench. And before him was a tall lawyer dressed in a gray pinstripe suit, with his back facing me. Being a connoisseur of premium-quality suits, I knew that the one worn by the lawyer was very expensive. The judge and the lawyer were discussing some issue, though I could not hear what they were saying. Both seemed very animated, with the judge moving his hands back and forth while the lawyer nodded. I took a few steps forward and sat down on one of the long wooden benches reserved for members of the public who wished to sit in on trials. I cast my eyes down to the ground.

"Not there, Mr. Sandersen—up here," commanded the judge, pointing to the seat normally reserved for prisoners.

"What have I done wrong?" I asked, struggling to maintain my composure. "A friend of mine asked me to meet him here at the courthouse at 9 A.M. As I walked up the steps, a police officer, Officer Perez, stopped me and escorted me into this courtroom. I have no idea what this is all about. My friend must be looking for me, and I'm feeling frustrated because I don't know why I've been asked to come in here. Have I been charged with some offence?"

"The crime of self-betrayal, amigo," stated the tall lawyer forcefully as he turned around and began to laugh. It was Julian! He rushed over and gave me the warmest hug he had ever given me. I glanced over at the judge who was laughing like a schoolchild.

"Hope we didn't scare you, Dar. Walter over here . . . I mean Judge Ford," Julian said, with a wink at his accomplice, "agreed to participate in this little charade to help me teach you about today's lesson. Walter and I used to spend a lot of time together when I was practicing law and we grew to be great friends. I called him up last night and asked him for a little favor," Julian explained with a smile.

Now the judge spoke up, addressing Julian with great affection and warmth. "You were the best lawyer I've ever met, Julian. No one could match your skills as a litigator. I truly have never encountered a better legal mind in my entire career on the bench. And I've seen some pretty brilliant lawyers in my time. But it's great to see you again, old friend. We all wondered where you had gone after you left your law practice. Pretty incredible story about your transformation up in the Himalayas—thanks for sharing it with me. The way you look now is going to take some getting used to. I mean, you're a young man again! Unbelievable—never seen or heard of anything like it. If you want to drop by for dinner any night, my door's always open for you, you know that, don't you, Julian?"

"I do. Thank you, Walter," responded Julian graciously.

"Julian, the whole legal community misses you. And as for you, Mr. Sandersen, I don't know what Julian over here is teaching you but I have a sense he's going to change your life."

"He already has, Sir. Already has," I responded, feeling more relaxed and finding the humor in Julian's endless shenanigans. I knew he liked to keep things interesting and shake things up.

The judge descended from his perch and gave Julian a two-armed handshake, the kind politicians on the campaign trail favor to show their warmth to voters. He then left the court-room from a private entrance in the back.

"Of course you have committed no offence, my friend. I know you left the stage of self-betrayal many weeks ago. I just wanted to do something that would bring the sixth of The 7 Stages of Self-Awakening to life for you. You see, the sixth stage is all about a trial."

"In a courtroom?"

"No, Dar, it's about a trial of a different sort. Before a seeker reaches the final destination of her biggest self, she will be presented with a trial. Before she reaches the treasure she has been longing for, she will be given a test. That's just the way life works on the path. If you study any great book of wisdom that describes this voyage of personal awakening, you will see that that seeker—or the hero—always faces some trial or adversity just before he gets the prize: the life he has always desired."

"Why does the world work in this way, Julian? Why are the laws of nature set up in such a way as to send the seeker a trial just before he gets to the end of his journey?"

"Good question. There are two reasons that nature sends a trial. First, it comes to ensure that the seeker has learned and fully integrated all the lessons he was meant to learn in his lifetime. And, second, it comes to test the resolve of the seeker. *Most people give up just before they reach their dreams. Most people quit only steps away from getting everything they wanted.* It's like the old story of the gold miner. He spent his entire life searching for the big nugget of gold that would make him a rich man. One day, as he was chipping away at a large piece of rock with his hammer, he decided he had had enough. Thirty-five years and he was still struggling to make ends meet. So he threw away the rock, laid down his hammer and left the mine forever. The next morning, a young man on his first day on the job picked up the large rock that the older miner had thrown away. He noted that much of the chipping had already been done so decided to take one good hard crack at it. Upon so doing, the young man could not believe what happened. The rock split in two, revealing the largest piece of gold any of the other miners had ever seen. The young man had struck it rich simply because the old miner had not had the wisdom and courage to persist until he got what he wanted.

Julian was speaking very passionately now. "'Adversity calls forth the soul's courage to bear unflinchingly whatever Heaven sends,' observed Euripides. You must *never ever give up when a trial presents itself on the path.* And many trials will present themselves along the way. Yes, before your greatest victory you will certainly face your greatest challenge. Just before you reach the *highest* point of your personal evolution, you can be sure you will face a *massive* test. That's what Stage Six speaks to. But having said that, before you receive some of the wins that you will earn by going deeper and deeper and remembering more of who you truly are, you will be sent many trials. With an awareness that this is all part of the route that you must travel to return home to your authentic self, it will be easier for you: you will be prepared."

"I understand. And you're right. Just knowing that I should expect some setbacks or that I will encounter some obstacles gives me a greater understanding of the way this process works. When the pitfalls do come up, I'll know that every other seeker on the path has experienced a similar kind of thing. That will make it easier. And I have a sense setbacks also come to strengthen me. Hard times do make us stronger people," I said. "Great suit, by the way," I added with a grin.

"I just borrowed it for the morning. Couldn't show up at this palace of justice without it. Coming back to this courthouse brings back so many memories. You know, amigo, I love my new life, the one I've lived since my return from India. I have never felt so comfortable in my own skin. I feel I am completely on-purpose and living the life I have been called to live. I wake up each morning with a splendid feeling of joy and boundless energy, eager to go out into the world and make something of the gifts and talents that have been granted to me. I really don't miss my old way of living much. It wasn't me. On the outside, I know it must have looked like I had it all. Gorgeous women around me, a jet-setting lifestyle, legal victories that were splashed over the front pages of the newspapers, more money than I knew what to do with. But, inside, I felt like a dead man walking. I had no spark. My internal light was dim. That was no way to live and, believe me, I do not miss that existence. But coming here today does bring back many memories. I made a lot of friends in the profession. And I met a lot of really good people. You know, Dar, *everyone* has goodness within them. When people act in mean or hurtful ways, don't make the mistake of believing that what you are seeing is an accurate representation of who they truly are. No one is bad at their core—they just *behave* in bad ways. I'm in no way saying that you need to remain around people who mistreat you. Of course you must set boundaries and protect yourself. I'm simply saying that you shouldn't fall for the illusion that there is such a thing as a bad human being. Those who do hurtful or vicious acts have been badly and viciously hurt by others. Don't make what they do about you, because it's not."

"I hear you, Julian. Interesting point. In our society, we rush to judgment on so many things. Someone does something we don't like and we instantly label them as 'bad' or 'ruthless' or 'selfish' or 'controlling.' What I understand you to be saying is that's a very superficial way of viewing the situation. We need to go deeper to discover the truth. Being a seeker is all about getting to the truth of what's really going on in a certain situation or in life in generally, isn't it?"

Julian nodded and smiled. He was happy with all that I was learning.

"And, at a deeper level, people who act in harsh ways are really doing nothing more that replaying the old tapes that have always run them. They are acting out the patterns and ways of behaving that they picked up in childhood, in an effort to cope and survive in the world. They don't know any better. Because they are asleep to what's going on for them internally, they blame the outside world for what's not working in their lives. In doing so, they never bring their own shadows,

shadows which run them, into the light of their conscious awareness. So they remain small and trapped in the lie that is their lives. And when people are taught a wiser and better way of doing things, they can begin to live a wiser and better life. When they realize that, in order for their lives to change, *they* must change, they wake up and begin to step towards their biggest lives."

Julian clapped his hands. He then got up on to the shining table in front of him and did a strange little dance. I was not sure if he learned that up in the Himalayas or from one of the other people that he coached. I had never seen anything like it. Julian saw me laughing but he didn't care. He just kept on waving his hands into the air and moving his feet from side to side. After a few minutes, he got down from the table and led me out of the courtroom.

"Let this courtroom and the mock trial I set up remind you of Stage Six of The 7 Stages of Self-Awakening. Before great things happen, sometimes, hard times occur. And please let my quirky little dance remind you that life's a game. Don't take it too seriously. Have fun. Dance. Laugh. Maintain a healthy dose of perspective. I know you have faced painful times in the recent past. I am sensitive to that. But I do invite you to remember that you have many many blessings in your life. Did you know that on the planet today, over one billion people will go to bed hungry tonight. There are children without food. There are people locked up and being tortured in prisons. There are other human beings—our brothers and sisters in this tribe called humanity—imprisoned in hospital rooms, struggling to survive the ravages of some disease. There are so many people who have far less than we do. And my heart cries out to them," said Julian, his tone softening. "I wish I could help each and every one of them. Remember what Mother Teresa said: 'There are no great acts, only small acts done with great love.'"

"She also said 'If I did not pick up that first person in Calcutta, I would not have picked up the forty-two thousand,'" I added. "I read that in one of the books I've been studying. And you are right, Julian. In the past, I always focused on what was missing in my life rather than on all the good I had. I guess maturity as a human being is loving what you have rather than worrying too much about having what you love. I know you believe we need to be proactive and chase our dreams. But I also hear you saying that bringing a deep sense of gratitude into one's life is important."

"Makes me think of that ancient Persian proverb: 'I cursed the fact I had no shoes until I saw a man who had no feet,'" noted Julian.

We left the courtroom in silence. Julian glanced at the paintings that lined the corridor as we walked towards the exit. On leaving the building, Julian stopped and looked out at the lush park across the street. He reached inside his suit jacket and handed me a piece of lined, legal-sized paper, the kind lawyers favor as they take their notes during court cases. On the top, it read: "Rules for Winning Trials."

"Here, amigo, this is for you," said Julian as he handed me the sheet of paper. "I'd like you to memorize these rules so that when challenging times appear on the path to awakening your biggest and best self, you'll have some specific ideas and tools to help you move through them." Julian paused and looked up to the sky. I heard him say the following words to no one in particular: "Please give me strength to be of greatest service."

He then looked at me once again. There was sadness in his eyes. "You are a powerful man," he said. "Only a few short months ago, you were ready to take your own life. But something within you wouldn't let you do it. Instead, you began letting life lead you, and began to be open to a new way of seeing things. This takes immense courage and speaks volumes about the person that you are. Since I have been coaching you, you have invested your trust in me and followed my instructions, strange as they appeared at times. You have gone deep, confronted your resistances, investigated your shadows and opened your heart. You are a good man in the process of becoming a great one, Dar. I so deeply feel that the world needs more people like you, more men and women who will heed the call of their hearts and awaken to their best lives. It breaks my heart to see people living at only a tiny fraction of their power and potential. It hurts me to see people acting in selfish ways, putting their own interests above those of others when they should be living in ways that help others *and* help themselves. Do you know how happy every person on the planet would feel if they made a little bit of time every day to be of greater service to others? Do you have any idea the joy that enters a person's being when they dedicate themselves to creating real and lasting value for other people? Helping other people get to their dreams is, when viewed from this frame of reference, a great gift you give yourself. But most people don't see this truth."

Julian became quiet.

"Most people are living with blindfolds over their eyes,

thinking that the world they are viewing is the only reality. You know that now. And they think that the mediocre and small lives they are leading are the only lives that are available to them. Each of our lives is destined to be great. That's part of the 'rough destiny' that has already been carved out for us. But it falls to us to build out the details of the destiny. It's that partnership I spoke of in an earlier coaching session. Life is a co-creative process. Do your best. Chase your dreams. Open your heart. Do your internal work. Take lots of action. Get up early and be disciplined. Do whatever is possible for you to do to close The Integrity Gap, stop recycling and realize The 4 Awakenings. Then—and only then—let go and accept what comes, knowing that it is what's best for you."

Julian's faith in the potential of human beings moved me. He was a believer in a society where too many people have given up the notion that each one of us can be great. Somewhere along the way, most of us bought into a lie that greatness was reserved for the chosen few. Somewhere along the way, some-one sold us a bill of goods that our lives were not meant to be extraordinary. Julian knew otherwise. He knew we were designed to play big. He understood we have been hardwired to shine brightly. He was awake to the truth that there are no extra people on the planet and we are all duty-bound to have an impact and bless the lives of those who surround us.

"I need to leave the city tomorrow. My next assignment is in England and I have a flight to catch at nine in the evening. I feel sad that I have to leave you, amigo. I am so very proud of what you have become and what you are growing into. And you deserve all that is happening for you. I offered the pathway and delivered the wisdom to you. But you had the bravery and good sense to execute the knowledge I shared. *Wisdom without execution is worthless.*"

I couldn't believe Julian was leaving. I had grown to love this man of few possessions who drove fast cars and sometimes donned fine suits. I had come to respect him enormously and care deeply for his welfare. And, to be honest, I noticed myself feeling a little afraid, now that I had learned I would be on my own, without a guide on the path. As always, Julian sensed what I was experiencing.

"You know you will never be alone, Dar. You now have Sasha. And you should know that as you venture farther along the path, you will naturally draw more seekers into your life. You will find more support along the way than you have ever imagined. Please do not worry. And also," Julian noted, "remember that, ultimately, all answers reside within you. You don't need a guide. This journey is not really about learning things you need to learn so much as it is about remembering things you have forgotten. The golden Buddha is already within you. All you need to do is remove the layers and all will be well in your universe."

"Thanks, Julian. I love you like a father, you know?"

"I know. Thank you. I'll be watching your star rise," he replied. "So let's meet tomorrow morning at five o'clock. I'd like you to meet me at the Rolling Hills Cemetery. I know you have questions about why we will be meeting there, but the answers will soon be apparent."

Julian gave me one of his trademark bear hugs and then walked slowly down the steps of the courthouse. I watched him say hello to a panhandler and then enter the park. Tears filled my eyes as I watched him. There would be a big hole in my life without Julian.

I glanced down at the paper in my hands. I read "Rules for Winning Trials"; there were seven of them and I knew they would be helpful in getting me through hard times. They read as follows:

**Rule #1:** Remember that life is a series of seasons. Every human being will have to endure the harshness of a few winters in order to get to the glory of the best summers. Never forget that winters do not last.

**Rule #2:** Join the Hope Club. Big, beautiful and seemingly impossible goals are superb vehicles to keep you inspired as you walk through adversity. I once quoted da Vinci's words to you: "Fix your course to a star and you can navigate any storm." When you are reaching for great and noble goals that speak to the best within you, your desire to reach them will pull you through the tough times that you will encounter along the seeker's path.

**Rule #3:** Keep in mind, at all times, that we grow the most from our greatest suffering. As we go through it, it hurts. But as we move through it, it also heals. When a jug of water falls to the floor and cracks, what was hidden within begins to pour out. When life sends you one if its curves, remember that it has come to help crack you open so that all the love, power and potential that had been slumbering within you can be poured into the world outside you. And, like a fractured bone, *we do become stronger in the broken places.*

**Rule #4:** Failure is a choice. Nothing can stop a man or a woman who simply refuses to be kept down. The book I mentioned—*The Go-Getter*—will be very helpful to you on this point. Read it often. Just make a decision from the center of your heart that, *no matter what happens to you,* you will keep walking the authentic path. Doing so will ensure you a life of *real* success.

**Rule #5:** During tough times, there is a tendency to let go of yourself. As you encounter adversity, have the discipline to maintain your routine. Get up early. Do your holy hour. Eat very well. Exercise. Spend time with nature and make sure that you do all you can to keep all four of your central dimensions—the mind, the body, the emotions and the spirit—in fine operating order.

**Rule #6:** Feel your feelings. When you are facing hard times, some people will tell you to "just think positive thoughts." Such advice is *not* helpful. While I agree that you cannot move the car forward if you are staring in the rearview mirror and that living in the past is unhealthy, one must not rush to reframe a so-called negative event as a positive one. Doing so will throw you into denial. Feel through the feelings of hurt, anger or sadness that will naturally surface. It's okay to be with them. It's actually healthy to do so. Processing through them allows you to release them. Just don't get stuck in them.

The key is really to strike a balance. Experience the feelings that arise so you do not end up swallowing them and allowing them to fester. At the same time, use your intellectual powers to see the silver lining that every dark cloud brings. This is not a scientific process and ultimately you need to do what feels right for you.

**Rule #7:** Remember that, no matter how hard things get, *you are never alone.*

I folded the paper. Julian's wisdom was profound as well as practical, although I wasn't quite sure of what he meant at the end about never being alone. I guessed that time and experience would bring the answer. Life was, I was discovering, the finest teacher.

I sat on those courthouse steps for an hour or more. I watched people walk by and birds soaring in the sky. I felt the rays of the sun on my face and a soft breeze wash through my hair. Julian would leave me tomorrow. My coach would be gone. He'd brought so much to my life. I vowed to begin giving back.

# CHAPTER 10

# The Seeker Awakens

*When you are inspired by some great purpose, some extraordinary project, all your thoughts break their bonds; your mind transcends limitations, your consciousness expands in every direction and you find yourself in a new, great and wonderful world. Dormant forces, faculties and talents become alive, and you discover yourself to be a greater person by far than you ever dreamed yourself to be.*

*—Patanjali*

The sun was rising as I drove out to the Rolling Hills Cemetery. This small and little-known cemetery was situated outside the city in a place known for its open spaces and beautiful meadows. Turning off the highway, I followed a winding road that took me past a lake where I used to fish with my father when I was a little boy.

As I drove up to the cemetery, I could hear loud chanting. As I came to a stop and got out of the car, I realized that someone was playing what appeared to be a Gregorian chant CD. With the chanting and the early morning fog still floating over the rolling hills, the whole environment took on a mystical air. Julian was nowhere to be seen.

I walked along the dirt path towards the small building that rested at the top of a grassy hill. As I headed up the slope, I stared out at the field of crosses and reflected on the lives that they stood for. More than ever, I realized that even the longest life is incredibly short when measured against the benchmark of eternity. We make so much of trivial things as we advance through life, forgetting what's most important and failing to appreciate that life will pass us by unless we get into the game. Often, by the time we wake up, it's too late and our best years have slipped away.

I had spent so much of my life chasing recognition and fortune. Yet no matter how much I achieved, it was never enough. It was almost like an addiction. Nothing could take the craving away and no matter how hard I tried to fight it, I was always pulled back in. Along the way, I had lost what meant most to me. I knew that I would never make that mistake again. Sure, outward success was important. I liked the fact that Julian's philosophy for personal fulfillment allowed for making money, having nice things and being "in the world." Actually, he suggested that such pursuits were very positive. We are spiritual beings but we live in a very human world and there was no reason to apologize for enjoying the material gifts this world presents to us. Julian's big idea was that chasing these kinds of fleeting rewards should not be the *main* aim of living. It truly was a matter of priorities and awakening my best self had to remain job number one.

As I neared the building, the chanting grew louder. I knew

that Julian was somewhere close by. This was, undoubtedly, another one of his unorthodox coaching scenarios. A smile appeared on my face.

"Julian," I called out. "I know you are here. Might as well tell me where you are."

There was no reply. I spoke more loudly. "Come on, Julian. I know you're up here. Where are you?"

Then I saw a figure approaching me through the mist. It was Julian and he was wearing his robe, with the hood covering his head. Both of his hands carried a bouquet of fresh flowers. On his back was his knapsack.

"Good morning, Dar," he said seriously. "I'll be leaving for the airport later today. But I needed to meet with you. This is our last coaching session together. I must share the final stage of The 7 Stages of Self-Awakening with you. Please follow me," Julian instructed as he led me away from the building and out into the field of tombstones. The chant music continued to play.

We walked for only a minute or so before Julian stopped at a freshly dug grave. He knelt down and encircled the gravesite with the fresh flowers he had been carrying. He was completely silent and appeared to be exceptionally respectful of the sacred place we were at.

"Julian, whose grave is this?" I asked softly.

"Yours," came the reply.

I had absolutely no idea what Julian meant by that comment. As we go through our days, people say things to us or act in certain ways. Much of the suffering we experience as human beings stems from the fact that we make certain assumptions about what happens to us. For example, we walk into work and a colleague does not say hello. We assume he is angry with us. That is our false assumption. The truth could be that his child is ill and he is preoccupied with that concern. The only way to test the truth of our assumptions is to have the courage to ask questions to clarify our understanding. This is nothing more than becoming good at communicating. But most people never do it. Over the past few weeks, I had committed to discovering the truth in all situations. I realized that, in the past, I had often misperceived certain situations and had decided to speak my truth when I needed more answers.

"Julian, what are you saying? How could this be my grave? I'm not dead. I've never been healthier or happier. I've never been so alive. What are you suggesting? I'm a little confused."

"Relax, amigo. This grave is a metaphor for the last lesson I have to share with you. This grave *could* be your grave. This grave could be *my* grave. It could be anyone's grave. The point is simply this: *in order to awaken to your best life, it's important that you die while you are alive.*"

"What do you mean by that?"

"Most people live as if they have all the time in the world. They wish they had more time in their days and yet they waste the time they have. They put off living until some event in the future occurs. Such people say 'I'll spend more time with my family once I get that big promotion' or 'I'll have more fun in life once my children grow up' or 'I'll chase my dreams once I make a little more money' or 'I'll improve my health as soon as I get through this stressful time.' *Life waits for no one.* One of the most important things I can teach you is to connect with your mortality on a regular basis. Remind yourself that time is your most precious commodity. Telling yourself that you will be your biggest self at some time in the future is presuming a lot. You, or I, could die today. As I told you when we met at The Q, none of us knows when our time is up. Every day should be lived as if it were the last day you had on the planet. Treat every one you meet as if you would never see them again. Take big risks as you move through your hours and seize all opportunities for personal greatness as they present themselves. I suggest that you get up nice and early every Sunday—or even every few Sundays—and come up here. Do it alone. Make it a regular ritual."

"And what exactly should I do once I get here?"

"Connect with your death. Think about the life you know you are capable of creating and remind yourself that you dishonor yourself if you don't live and breathe it each day. Every single moment above ground is a giant opportunity. I told you that, Dar. Every single day you wake up is a gift to be celebrated. You are destined to shine. Come here to reconnect with the delicacy of life. Just think about it: some of the people on the planet who will wake up today will be dead by the time the sun sets. Most of them will not imagine that such a thing is about to happen to them. They had all these great plans for when the time was right. *No one ever plans to die.*"

That last phrase hit me hard. I knew I was living more consciously and with a greater sense of joy and enthusiasm than I had ever experienced. But I was still holding back. I was still holding back some of my love from Sasha. I could be so much more for her. And as I reflected more deeply, I realized that behind that resistance was fear. I feared that if I completely opened my heart to her, I could be hurt or perhaps taken advantage of. My fear had no basis in reality—Sasha was an incredible woman, in all respects. But fears often have no basis in reality; they are merely illusions we set up. And they truly are only six inches deep.

I had also been playing smaller than I should have been with my children. I knew I could become an extraordinary father and, in that moment, I made a self-promise to do so. The more I thought about it, the more I came to see that there was so much more that I could do and be. Why couldn't I be one of the greatest leaders in my industry? Why couldn't I add incredible value to hundreds if not thousands of lives? Why couldn't I get closer to the state of personal enlightenment than I had ever imagined myself getting to?

"Do you remember the exercise I asked you to do the time we met at the schoolhouse?" asked Julian.

"How could I forget?" I asked. "You asked me to write my obituary. You requested that I write out the story of my life so that I would have the wisdom and the awareness to live my life backwards. By knowing where I dreamed of being at the end, I could make the choices required in every moment of every hour of every day to get me there."

"Perfectly said."

"And I often read my obituary aloud during my morning holy hour. Right after I wake up, it's generally one of the first things I do. That single act alone has made a profound difference in the way I think, feel and act during my days."

"That leads me elegantly to the seventh and final stage of the process of self-awakening. After you leave the lie that your life once was by deciding to embark upon the path of the truth at The Choicepoint..."

"Stages One and Two of the process," I interjected.

"Correct. Well, after you move through those first two stages you get to the third stage which is where you begin to see through a new set of eyes. You begin to discover the truth. You realize how much power has been sleeping within you. You begin to grow in awareness as to how you have been betraying and limiting yourself. You start to see how wonderful this world of ours is and how much joy is waiting for you. What comes next, amigo?" Julian asked.

"Stage Four. This is where, as the seeker advances along the path, he or she hungers for answers to the many questions that begin to surface. At this stage, the seeker looks for guides and masters to help him find his way. All the new learning and heightened awareness that the seeker is receiving then leads to confusion."

"Yes. The very foundations upon which the seeker has stood begin to crumble. All the beliefs and assumptions about the way the world works and how he occurs within it are being questioned and re-evaluated. Stage Five is a time of enormous upheaval and change. It's also a time of very beautiful personal growth. The caterpillar may be experiencing the darkness of the cocoon, but guess what's really happening?"

"A butterfly is being born," I replied confidently.

"You got it. *It's all good.* Next comes the inevitable trial that every seeker on the path will experience. Just before great victory, life always sends the traveler a big test. How we respond at such times in many ways defines our destinies.

Choosing to be courageous and pressing forward is your best move. And this, of course brings me to the final stage, The Great Awakening of Self. You have experienced pieces of every stage during the time we have been together. Yes, I have manufactured some scenarios for you so that each part of the process would come to life. I did this to help you learn and grow in your understanding. But a lot of what you experienced came organically. As you left the lie and made the choice to wake up, you yourself turned to books and guides to help you learn and build your base of wisdom. And as you did, you yourself experienced the confusion and transformation that Stage Five presents. And because you did not give up, *real* transformation has occurred in your life. It all looks very different than it did just a while ago, doesn't it?"

"No doubt. My life has become beautiful, Julian. I've never been happier. I am so grateful to you."

"You are most welcome, Dar. And after I leave, life will bring you its own scenarios and experiences and you will go through some of the stages without my being around. Life will become your coach and best teacher—if you'll let it."

Julian rubbed one of his hands along the embroidery on his robe.

"Stage Seven is the final destination. To get completely to this point on the path is to become enlightened. As I've mentioned, few have reached this lofty place. But that will change. I want you to help me by spreading my philosophy to all those whose lives you touch. I have a strong sense that you want to give something back to me for what I've given you. Please know that I have no need for any worldly things. Sure I had fun driving my old Ferrari and wearing that splendid suit at the courthouse. But they are not what's most important to me. I want to change the world, my friend. I want to have an impact on as many people as I possibly can. I was an unhappy lawyer, struggling in life—spiritually speaking. My life was completely out of balance and dramatically out of control. But just look at me now," Julian said excitedly. "What I learned up in those mountains works and I want every single person I have the opportunity to affect to discover what I uncovered up there with those enlightened sages. The only thing I ask you to do is to tell others about what I've shared with you. The best way to learn is to teach, so you'll be doing yourself a favor in the process."

Julian walked over to me and put both his hands on my shoulders. He looked up into the blue sky a final time. He closed his eyes.

"Dar, you have been an excellent student. I couldn't be happier for you, in terms of the way things look in your life today. You are headed to magnificent places and you cannot imagine the wonders that are awaiting you. I have enjoyed our time together enormously. You have treated me with great kindness, respect and love. Please continue to keep listening to that little voice that's growing within you. It's the call of your heart and, if you keep trusting it, it will lead you to where you need to go. Keep letting the talents you've been given see the light of day. Continue to create value for everyone in your life. And keep walking this path, no matter what things may come up. In so doing, your life will be a great one and your legacy will be large."

Julian opened his eyes. A single tear ran down his cheek and onto his robe. He looked down at the spot it made and laughed.

"Every ending is a new beginning. You taught me that a while ago—don't forget it, coach," I said playfully.

"Well said, amigo. It's just that it's hard for me to leave the people I've grown to love. You, and the rest of the people I've coached since I returned from India, are my heroes. The bravery you all show humbles me. I wish I could remain here and guide you along the path. But that's not what you need. And that's not what I'm destined to do. Before I leave, I want to do something, if I may?" asked Julian.

"Of course, Julian, anything you want to do is fine with me."

Julian took off his knapsack and opened it up. He pulled out a worn, leather-bound journal and opened it up to a particular page. Standing at the edge of the grave, and speaking in a strong, loud voice, Julian said: "I want to do something I've never done. I want to read my obituary aloud." He then paused before he spoke the following words:

### The Obituary of Julian Mantle

*Julian Mantle was a man who believed in the power of the human spirit to be a force for good on the planet. He was an idealist and a person who truly believed that every person alive could make a genuine difference if they chose to accept the call on their lives to do so.*

*Julian was a simple man. He loved great books, sunsets, star-filled nights and a thick piece of chocolate cake every once in a while. Most of all, Julian loved people and spent his life helping them discover who they truly are.*

*He made a lot of mistakes in his time. But he learned from them. He encountered much personal pain, but he grew from it.*

*Julian never ran from his fears. Instead, he ran to them, and in so doing, he reclaimed his freedom. He was authentic, courageous and loving.*

*Julian died last night, at the tender age of 108. He touched many lives and his presence will be missed.*

On hearing Julian's words, I began to cry. When I looked up, I saw that he was gone. I looked across the field but Julian was nowhere to be seen. The chanting could still be heard from the small building on the hill, and the sun was shining brightly. There was not a single cloud in the sky.

As I made my way past the tombstones, something sparkled amidst the grass. I bent down and was stunned by what I saw. It was a small golden Buddha that had been attached to a long, thin piece of leather so that it could be worn around the neck. On the back of the carefully crafted object were the following simple words, written in a tiny script:

*Awaken Best Self and Keep Shining.*
*With love, JM*

I put Julian's gift around my neck and walked towards my car. I couldn't stop smiling. My life had become beautiful.

# The 7 Stages of
# Self-Awakening

**STAGE 1: Living a Lie** (The Stage of Self-Betrayal)

**STAGE 2: The Choicepoint** (The Stage of Releasing Control and Breaking Your Chains)

**STAGE 3: Awareness of Wonder and Possibility** (The Stage of Seeing with New Eyes)

**STAGE 4: Instruction from Masters** (The Stage of Learning, Failing and Preparation)

**STAGE 5: Transformation and Rebirth** (The Stage of Emptying and Refilling)

**STAGE 6: The Trial** (The Stage of Testing and Confirmation)

**STAGE 7: The Great Awakening of Self** (The Stage of Fearlessness)

# The 5 Daily Devotions

1. Rise each and every morning at 5 A.M. Those who get up early are those who get the best from life.
2. Set aside the first sixty minutes of your day as your "holy hour." This is your sacred time to do the inner work (prayer, meditation, journaling, reading from the wisdom literature, reflecting on the state of your life) that will help you live your highest life.
3. Display a standard of care, compassion and character well beyond what anyone could ever imagine from you. In doing so, you will be doing your part to aid in the building of a new world.
4. Display a standard of excellence at work far higher than anyone would ever expect from you. Abundance and fulfillment will flow back to you.
5. Devote yourself to being the most loving person you know and thinking, feeling and acting as though you are one of the greatest people currently on the planet (because you are). Your life will never be the same and you will bless many lives.

## ABOUT ROBIN SHARMA

Robin Sharma is one of the world's premier experts on leadership, elite performance and self-discovery. He is the author of numerous bestsellers, including the #1 international bestseller *The Monk Who Sold His Ferrari*, its popular sequels *Leadership Wisdom from The Monk Who Sold His Ferrari* and *Family Wisdom from The Monk Who Sold His Ferrari, Who Will Cry When You Die?* and *The Saint, The Surfer & The CEO*, a #1 bestseller at amazon.com. A frequent guest of the national media, Robin has starred in his own PBS special and appeared on over 1,000 television and radio shows. He is also in high demand across the globe as a keynote speaker and frequently shares the stage with such individuals as Jack Welch, Bill Clinton, Christopher Reeve, Dr. Phil, Deepak Chopra and Wayne Dyer.

A former lawyer who holds two law degrees, one of them a masters, Robin is the visionary CEO of Sharma Leadership International (SLI), a widely respected learning services firm that helps employees and entrepreneurs realize their highest professional and personal potential. SLI also runs the highly acclaimed *Elite Performers Series*™, a strikingly effective 2-day coaching process that helps individuals show excellence in all they do, and *The Monthly Coach*™ program, Robin's Book and CD of the Month club. As well, Robin is a top executive/life coach to CEOs, entrepreneurs and some of the planet's most successful people.

Robin's personal mission is to help people rediscover who they truly are and live in a way that creates value for others. Through *The Robin Sharma Foundation for Children*, he helps underprivileged children stand up for their dreams.

For more information on Robin Sharma or any of SLI's learning products, please visit **robinsharma.com** or call 1.888.RSHARMA (774.2762).

# THE SHARMA LEADERSHIP REPORT

Free subscription offer to pur-
chasers of this book for a limited
time only (annual subscription has a
$95 value).

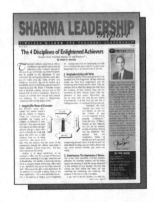

*The Sharma Leadership Report*,
Robin Sharma's widely read elec-
tronic newsletter, is packed with
practical wisdom, lessons and tools
that will help you live your biggest
life, personally, professionally and spiritually. People from
around the world and from all walks of life read this highly
inspirational report to help them balance work and family,
achieve elite performance, manage stress, deepen relationships and live their dreams. It is a very special publication
and one that will help you enormously.

To order your free subscription, simply visit **robinsharma.com**
and register online today. We also invite you to share this elec-
tronic newsletter with your friends, so that they too will
receive powerful ideas to live greatly and leave a legacy.

## KEYNOTES AND SEMINARS
## WITH ROBIN SHARMA

Robin Sharma is one of the world's most sought-after professional speakers on leadership, elite performance, managing change and personal discovery. His pioneering insights on these topics have made him the first choice of organizations seeking a high-profile keynote speaker or seminar leader whose message will transform lives, create tangible results and restore commitment and productivity in these uncertain times. Robin's extraordinarily inspirational presentations are fully customized through a unique research process, rich in practical content that your people can use immediately, and carefully designed to help individuals move to all-new levels of performance, passion, creativity and individual fulfillment.

To book Robin Sharma for your next conference or in-house seminar, visit **robinsharma.com** or contact:

Marnie Ballane
VP of Speaking Services
Sharma Leadership International
Tel: 1.888.RSHARMA (774.2762)
e-mail: marnie@robinsharma.com

# PERSONAL COACHING SERVICES
## WITH ROBIN SHARMA

1. *The Monthly Coach*®
   *The Monthly Coach* is Robin's highly acclaimed Book and
   CD of the Month club. Every 30 days, you receive one of
   the most powerful books available on personal develop-
   ment, leadership, relationships or business success, along
   with a CD that contains Robin's summary of the book's
   best points and his coaching insights/tactics on how to
   translate the book's knowledge into real results that will
   make you more successful, more fulfilled and happier. To
   register, simply visit robinsharma.com today.

2. *Awakening Best Self Weekend*™ *(ABS)*
   This is Robin's 2½-day personal transformation program
   that has helped people from across the globe rediscover
   their biggest lives and live with all-new levels of joy, abundance, love and fulfillment. *ABS* weekend has been called
   one of the most effective self-discovery processes on the
   market today, and attendees have found that the experience has helped them release fears, break through limitations, reconnect with their authentic power and live the
   lives they have always dreamed of. Participants have come
   from all over the world, including the United States,
   Mexico, the United Kingdom, Europe and Canada. To
   register for the next ABS weekend and to read recent
   testimonials, visit robinsharma.com or e-mail us at
   coaching@robinsharma.com.

3. *The Elite Performers Series™ (EPS)*

*The Elite Performers Series* is Sharma Leadership International's flagship corporate coaching program, which is designed to transform employees into elite performers who lead their field. Participants can expect to dramatically boost productivity, creativity, passion, commitment and play a far higher game professionally as well as personally. The testimonials confirming the power of the EPS (which you can view at robinsharma.com) say it all. For upcoming dates or to have *The Elite Performers Series* in-house for your organization, simply visit robinsharma.com or e-mail us at coaching@robinsharma.com.

4. *The Masters Series™*

Each year, schedule permitting, Robin Sharma accepts up to 5 clients in this very exclusive, world-class, weekly coaching program. Over the course of a full year, Robin will serve as your personal executive/life coach, working with you to help take your business to previously unimagined levels of success, as well as help you create your highest life professionally, physically, personally and spiritually. Previous clients have experienced transformative results.

For more information on these personal coaching services, visit robinsharma.com or contact:

Al Moscardelli
Vice President of Coaching Services
Sharma Leadership International
Tel: 1.888.RSHARMA (774.2762)
e-mail: coaching@robinsharma.com

# S P E C I A L    O F F E R

Order these selected Thorsons and Element titles direct from the publisher and receive £1 off each title! Visit www.thorsonselement.com for additional special offers.

Free post and packaging for UK delivery (overseas and Ireland, £2.00 per book).

| | |
|---|---|
| **The Monk Who Sold His Ferrari**<br>Robin Sharma (0007179731) | £7.99 retail – £1 = £6.99 |
| **The Alchemist**<br>Paulo Coelho (0722532938) | £7.99 retail – £1 = £6.99 |
| **Liberation**<br>Barefoot Doctor (0007165102) | £7.99 retail – £1 = £6.99 |
| **The Journey**<br>Brandon Bays (0722538391) | £10.99 retail – £1 = £9.99 |

Place your order by post, phone, fax, or email, listed below. Be certain to quote reference code **714N** to take advantage of this special offer.

Mail Order Dept. (REF: **714N**)           Email: customerservices@harpercollins.co.uk
HarperCollins*Publishers*                                    Phone: 0870 787 1724
Westerhill Road                                                    Fax: 0870 787 1725
Bishopbriggs G64 2QT

Credit cards and cheques are accepted. Do not send cash. Prices shown above were correct at time of press. Prices and availability are subject to change without notice.

BLOCK CAPITALS PLEASE

Name of cardholder _____

Address of cardholder _____

_____

_____

Postcode _____

Delivery address (if different)

_____

_____

_____

Postcode _____

I've enclosed a cheque for £_____, made payable to HarperCollins*Publishers*, or please charge my Visa/MasterCard/Switch (circle as appropriate)

Card Number: _____

Expires: __/__                     Issue No: __/__                     Start Date: __/__
Switch cards need an issue number or start date validation.

Signature:_____

**thorsons**
**element**

# Make
# www.thorsonselement.com
# your online sanctuary

Get online information, inspiration and
guidance to help you on the path to physical
and spiritual well-being. Drawing on the integrity
and vision of our authors and titles, and with
health advice, articles, astrology, tarot, a
meditation zone, author interviews and events
listings, www.thorsonselement.com is a great
alternative to help create space and peace
in our lives.

So if you've always wondered about practising
yoga, following an allergy-free diet, using the
tarot or getting a life coach, we can point you
in the right direction.

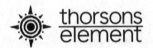

thorsons
element